Thoracic Anatomy, Part II: Pleura, Mediastinum, Diaphragm, Esophagus

Guest Editor

JEAN DESLAURIERS, MD, FRCS(C)

THORACIC SURGERY CLINICS

www.thoracic.theclinics.com

Consulting Editor

MARK K. FERGUSON, MD

May 2011 • Volume 21 • Number 2

SAUNDERS an imprint of ELSEVIER, Inc.

W.B. SAUNDERS COMPANY
A Division of Elsevier Inc.

1600 John F. Kennedy Boulevard • Suite 1800 • Philadelphia, Pennsylvania 19103-2899

http://www.theclinics.com

THORACIC SURGERY CLINICS Volume 21, Number 2
May 2011 ISSN 1547-4127, ISBN-13: 978-1-4377-2269-7

Editor: Barbara Cohen-Kligerman
Developmental Editor: Donald Mumford

Thoracic Surgery Clinics (ISSN 1547-4127) is published quarterly by Elsevier Inc., 360 Park Avenue South, New York, NY 10010-1710. Months of publication are February, May, August, and November. Business and editorial offices: 1600 John F. Kennedy Boulevard, Suite 1800, Philadelphia, PA 19103-2899. Periodicals postage paid at New York, NY, and additional mailing offices. Subscription prices are $295.00 per year (US individuals), $385.00 per year (US institutions), $141.00 per year (US Students), $367.00 per year (Canadian individuals), $487.00 per year (Canadian institutions), $192.00 per year (Canadian and foreign students), $391.00 per year (foreign individuals), and $487.00 per year (foreign institutions). Foreign air speed delivery is included in all Clinics' subscription prices. All prices are subject to change without notice. **POSTMASTER:** Send address changes to Thoracic Surgery Clinics, Elsevier Health Sciences Division, Subscription Customer Service, 3251 Riverport Lane, Maryland Heights, MO 63043. **Customer Service (orders, claims, online, change of address): Telephone: 1-800-654-2452 (U.S. and Canada); 314-447-8871 (outside U.S. and Canada). Fax: 314-447-8029. Email: journalscustomerservice-usa@elsevier.com (for print support); journalsonlinesupport-usa@elsevier.com (for online support).**

Reprints. For copies of 100 or more, of articles in this publication, please contact Commercial Rights Department, Elsevier Inc., 360 Park Avenue South, New York, NY 10010-1710. Tel: (212) 633-3812; Fax: (212) 462-1935; E-mail: reprints@elsevier.com.

Thoracic Surgery Clinics is covered in *MEDLINE/PubMed (Index Medicus)* and *EMBASE/Excerpta Medica.*

Printed and bound by CPI Group (UK) Ltd, Croydon, CR0 4YY

Transferred to Digital Print 2011

Contributors

CONSULTING EDITOR

MARK K. FERGUSON, MD
Professor of Surgery, Section of Cardiac and
Thoracic Surgery, The University of Chicago
Medical Center, Chicago, Illinois

GUEST EDITOR

JEAN DESLAURIERS, MD, FRCS(C)
Professor of Surgery, Laval University;
Thoracic Surgeon, Institut Universitaire de
Cardiologie et de Pneumologie de Québec,
Quebec City, Quebec, Canada

AUTHORS

SHAHAB A. AKHTER, MD
Associate Professor of Surgery, Section
of Cardiac and Thoracic Surgery, The
University of Chicago, Chicago, Illinois

FAWAZ ALTAF, MB, ChB, FRCS(C), FRCS(I)
Surgical Fellow, Division of Thoracic Surgery,
Department of Surgery, McMaster University,
St Joseph's Healthcare, Hamilton, Ontario,
Canada

CESAR ARAUJO, MD
Department of Radiology, Federal University
of Bahia School of Medicine, Salvador-Ba,
Brazil

W. FREDERICK BENNETT, BSc, MD, FRCS(C)
Assistant Professor, Division of Thoracic
Surgery, Department of Surgery, McMaster
University, St Joseph's Healthcare, Hamilton,
Ontario, Canada

FRANÇOIS BERTIN, MD
Service de Chirurgie Thoracique et
Cardiovasculaire, CHU Dupuytren, Limoges,
France

JEAN-PHILIPPE BOLDUC, MD
Department of Radiology, Institut Universitaire
de Cardiologie et de Pneumologie de Québec,
Canada

MARY P. BRONNER, MD
Professor of Pathology, Cleveland Clinic Lerner
College of Medicine of Case Western Reserve
University; Director, GI Pathology; Section
Head, Molecular Morphologic Pathology,
Department of Anatomic Pathology,
Cleveland Clinic, Cleveland, Ohio

FRANÇOIS DAGENAIS, MD, FRCS(C)
Department of Cardiac Surgery, Institut
Universitaire de Cardiologie et de Pneumologie
de Laval, Laval Hospital, Quebec, Canada

GAIL E. DARLING, MD, FACS, FRCSC
Professor of Thoracic Surgery, Kress Family
Chair in Esophageal Cancer, Toronto General
Hospital, University of Toronto, Toronto,
Ontario, Canada

STEVEN R. DEMEESTER, MD
Associate Professor, Department of Surgery,
Keck School of Medicine, University of
Southern California, Los Angeles, California

JEAN DESLAURIERS, MD, FRCS(C)
Professor of Surgery, Laval University;
Thoracic Surgeon, Institut Universitaire de
Cardiologie et de Pneumologie de Québec,
Quebec City, Quebec, Canada

CAO DIANBO, MD
Department of Radiology, First Teaching
Hospital of Jilin University, Changchun, Jilin
Province, People's Republic of China

ROBERT DOWNEY, MD, FACS
Thoracic Service, Department of Surgery,
Memorial Sloan-Kettering Cancer Center,
New York, New York

DAVID J. FINLEY, MD
Thoracic Service, Department of Surgery,
Memorial Sloan-Kettering Cancer Center,
New York, New York

HAMID HEMATTI, MD
Research Fellow, Department of Thoracic
and Cardiovascular Surgery, The University
of Texas MD Anderson Cancer Center,
Houston, Texas

KLAUS LOUREIRO IRION, MD, PhD, FRCR
Department of Radiology, Liverpool Heart
and Chest Hospital, The Royal Liverpool and
Broadgreen University Hospital, Liverpool,
United Kingdom

SHAF KESHAVJEE, MD, MSc, FRCSC, FACS
Surgery-in-Chief, Toronto General Hospital,
University Health Network; Professor, Division
of Thoracic Surgery, University of Toronto,
Toronto, Ontario, Canada

JI LI, MD
Heilongjian Provincial Hospital, Haerbin,
People's Republic of China

CHEN LIANG, MD
Director, Department of Radiology, First
Teaching Hospital of Jilin University,
Changchun, Jilin Province, People's Republic
of China

RICHARD W. LIGHT, MD
Division of Allergy, Pulmonary and Critical Care
Medicine, Department of Medicine, Vanderbilt
University Medical Center, Nashville,
Tennessee

GUOJIN LIU, MD
Professor of Surgery, Jilin University, First
Teaching Hospital, Changchun, Jilin Province,
People's Republic of China

WEI LIU, MD
Assistant Director, Thoracic Surgical Service,
First Teaching Hospital of Jilin University,
Changchun, Changchun, Jilin Province,
People's Republic of China

REZA J. MEHRAN, MD
Professor, Department of Thoracic and
Cardiovascular Surgery, The University
of Texas MD Anderson Cancer Center,
Houston, Texas

ARZU OEZCELIK, MD
Department of Surgery, Keck School of
Medicine, University of Southern California,
Los Angeles, California

SERGIO TADEU PEREIRA, MD
Department of Thoracic Surgery, Santa
Casa De Misericordia Hospital,
Praça Cons Almeida Couto, Centro
Medico Celso Figueroa, Nazaré,
Salvador-Ba, Brazil

THOMAS W. RICE, MD
Professor of Surgery, Cleveland Clinic Lerner
College of Medicine of Case Western Reserve
University; Section Head, Thoracic Surgery,
Department of Thoracic and Cardiovascular
Surgery; The Daniel and Karen Lee Endowed
Chair in Thoracic Surgery, Cleveland Clinic,
Cleveland, Ohio

VALERIE W. RUSCH, MD
Thoracic Service, Department of Surgery,
Memorial Sloan-Kettering Cancer Center,
New York, New York

NAJIB SAFIEDDINE, MD, FRCSC
Resident, Division of Thoracic Surgery, Toronto
General Hospital, University of Toronto,
Toronto, Ontario, Canada

CARLA M. SEVIN, MD
Division of Allergy, Pulmonary and Critical Care
Medicine, Department of Medicine, Vanderbilt
University Medical Center, Nashville,
Tennessee

LI SHUANG, MD
Department of Radiology, First Teaching
Hospital of Jilin University, Changchun,
Jilin Province, People's Republic of China

SHONA E. SMITH, MD, FRCSC
Thoracic Surgery Fellow, Division of Thoracic
Surgery, Toronto General Hospital, University
of Toronto, Toronto, Ontario, Canada

PAULA A. UGALDE, MD
Assistant Professor, Department of
Thoracic Surgery, Santa Casa De
Misericordia Hospital, Praça Cons Almeida
Couto, Centro Medico Celso Figueroa,
Nazaré, Salvador-Ba, Brazil

JINGYI WANG, MD
Heilongjian Provincial Hospital, Haerbin;
Professor of Surgery, Jilin University, First
Teaching Hospital, Changchun, Jilin Province,
People's Republic of China

LIU WEI, MD
Associate Director, Department of Thoracic
Surgery, First Teaching Hospital of Jilin
University, Changhun, Jilin Province, People's
Republic of China

SIONA E. SMITH, MD, FRCSC
Cardiac Surgery Fellow, Division of Thoracic Surgery, Toronto General Hospital, University of Toronto, Toronto, Ontario, Canada

PAULA A. UGALDE, MD
Assistant Professor, Department of Thoracic Surgery, Santa Casa De Misericordia Hospital Prof Cons Almeida Couto, Centro Medico Celso Figueroa, Hozana, Salvador-Ba, Brazil

JINGYI WANG, MD
Heilongjian Provincial Hospital, Harbin; Professor of Surgery, Jilin University, First Teaching Hospital, Changchun, Jilin Province, People's Republic of China

LIU WEI, MD
Associate Director, Department of Thoracic Surgery, First Teaching Hospital of Jilin University, Changchun, Jilin Province, People's Republic of China

Contents

abnormal anatomy with imaging characteristics provides additional information that can be useful not only to accurately locate pleuropulmonary lesions but also to characterize abnormalities, such as pleural thickening or malignant processes.

The Mediastinum

Having a clear understanding of the divisions of the mediastinum is important for the thoracic surgeon who daily has to establish a differential diagnosis of mediastinal masses based on their location, as well as to select the best surgical approach to access the mediastinum to obtain diagnostic material, to drain mediastinal spaces, or to excise mediastinal tumors. In this respect, the most useful classifications appear to be the 3-compartment model and Shields' 3-zone classification. This article describes the various classifications of the mediastinum.

In the case of the thymus gland, the most common indications for resection are myasthenia gravis or thymoma. The consistency and appearance of the thymus gland make it difficult at times to discern from mediastinal fatty tissues. Having a clear understanding of the anatomy and the relationship of the gland to adjacent structures is important.

The venous side of the systemic vascular circulation returns the left ventricular cardiac output in a converging fashion to the superior and inferior vena cava and hence to the right atrium. Oxygenated blood is returned to the left atrium. The volumes of these 2 systems are in balance in a normal physiologic state.

This article describes the normal anatomy of the heart and pericardium. Included is a detailed description of the pericardium, mediastinal nerves, cardiac chambers, valves, coronary arteries and veins, and the conduction tissues. As cardiac and thoracic surgery continue to get more specialized and the procedures become less invasive, it is essential for the cardiothoracic surgeon to have a thorough working knowledge of cardiothoracic anatomy.

For a surgeon performing chest operation, thorough knowledge of the anatomy of the thoracic aorta and of its branches are essential not only to ensure the preservation of adequate organ vascular supply during reconstructive surgery of the esophagus or trachea but also to avoid injury to important thoracic vascular structures. This knowledge is of paramount importance especially for surgeons performing operations for mediastinal disorders or tumors to avoid catastrophic complications. This article discusses the anatomy and the most common congenital abnormalities of the thoracic aorta and its branches.

Anatomy of the Thoracic Duct 229

Hamid Hematti and Reza J. Mehran

The thoracic duct is a major anatomic structure of the upper part of the abdomen, chest, and the lower part of the neck. This article reviews the embryology, anatomy, and multiple variations of the thoracic duct. Proper knowledge of this anatomy should ease understanding the pathophysiology of diseases involving the lymph channels and also prevent injury to the duct during major procedures in which the duct or its tributaries can be involved.

Nerves of the Mediastinum 239

Jingyi Wang, Ji Li, Guojin Liu, and Jean Deslauriers

Knowledge of the anatomy of the mediastinal nerves is essential for the evaluation and surgical treatment of most thoracic neoplasms. Thorough knowledge of the normal anatomy of the mediastinal nerves and of their variants cannot be overestimated because nerve trauma during nerve anatomy is also important because mediastinal or lung tumors can locally infiltrate those nerves either directly or through nodal metastases, making them generally unresectable.

Correlative Anatomy for the Mediastinum 251

Paula A. Ugalde, Sergio Tadeu Pereira, Cesar Araujo, and Klaus Loureiro Irion

Diseases of the mediastinum comprise a wide spectrum of benign and malignant entities that share the same anatomic site within the chest. Correct management often requires a multidisciplinary approach. Diagnostic imaging modalities such as computed tomography (CT), magnetic resonance imaging (MRI), ultrasonography, and positron emission tomography play a major role in the diagnosis of mediastinal diseases and in guiding minimally invasive diagnostic procedures, minimizing the risk of imaging-guided biopsies. This article describes the mediastinal anatomy, correlating the findings of plain radiography, CT, and MRI.

The Diaphragm

Anatomy of the Normal Diaphragm 273

Robert Downey

The thoracic diaphragm is a dome-shaped septum, composed of muscle surrounding a central tendon, which separates the thoracic and abdominal cavities. The function of the diaphragm is to expand the chest cavity during inspiration and to promote occlusion of the gastroesophageal junction. This article provides an overview of the normal anatomy of the diaphragm.

Correlative Anatomy of the Diaphragm 281

Cao Dianbo, Liu Wei, Jean-Philippe Bolduc, and Jean Deslauriers

The diaphragm acts as a partition between the thoracic and abdominal cavities. On computed tomography, it is seen as a curved soft-tissue density with fat below and aerated lung above. The direct multiplanar capability of magnetic resonance technology can improve depiction of normal or abnormal diaphragmatic anatomy. Despite the usefulness of these imaging modalities, adequate visualization of the diaphragm can be difficult. Thoracic surgeons must be familiar with the correlative anatomy of the diaphragm because this knowledge is a prerequisite to making an accurate diagnosis of diaphragmatic abnormalities.

The Esophagus

Thoracic Surgery Clinics

VISIT THE CLINICS ONLINE!

Access your subscription at:
www.theclinics.com

Thoracic Surgery Clinics

FORTHCOMING ISSUES

August 2011

From Residency to Retirement: Building
a Successful Thoracic Surgery Career
Sean Grondin, MD, and F.G. Pearson, MD,
Guest Editors

November 2011

Benign Esophageal Diseases
Blair Jobe, Guest Editor

February 2012

Current Management Guidelines in Thoracic
Surgery
Blair Marshall, MD, Guest Editor

RECENT ISSUES

February 2011

Thymoma
Federico Venuta, MD, Guest Editor

November 2010

Chest Wall Surgery
Gaetano Rocco, MD, Guest Editor

August 2010

Air Leak after Pulmonary Resection
Alessandro Brunelli, MD, Guest Editor

ISSUE OF RELATED INTEREST

Radiologic Clinics of North America Volume 48, Issue 1 (January 2010),
Thoracic MDCT Comes of Age
Sanjeev Bhalla, MD, Guest Editor

VISIT THE CLINICS ONLINE

Access your subscription at:
www.theclinics.com

Preface
Thoracic Anatomy: Pleura and Pleural Spaces, Mediastinum, Diaphragm, and Esophagus

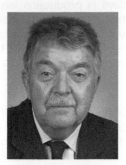

Jean Deslauriers, MD, FRCS(C)
Guest Editor

In the preface of his masterpiece *"De Humani Corporis Fabrica"* (1543), Andreas Vesalius (1514–1564) wrote that anatomy should be regarded as the firm foundation of the art of medicine and its essential preliminary. This observation, which marked a new era in the history of medicine, is even more applicable to surgery, where safe techniques are dependent on adequate knowledge and understanding of normal anatomy. Although thoracic anatomy remains the same as it was in the past, our understanding of it is vastly different that what it was only 10 or 20 years ago. This relates to new imaging techniques (CT, MR, echo), which have given us new visions of the morphology of thoracic organs, and to new surgical techniques, which use the smallest of incisions to achieve the same objectives previously accomplished through open thoracotomies. Ultimately, successful surgical work without well-founded knowledge of topographical and sectional anatomy is not possible, and all surgeons need an atlas of thoracic anatomy that can be referenced when needed. The growing recognition of the important relationship between the art of surgery and success in surgical therapies reemphasizes the value of intimate knowledge of anatomy.

This issue of *Thoracic Surgery Clinics* is the second of two parts devoted to the study of thoracic anatomy. It is written by surgeons who possess detailed knowledge of a particular segment of anatomy – whether it is the pleura, mediastinum, diaphragm, or esophagus – who can comprehend it, and who are able to establish structural, functional, and imaging relationships. Together these two issues of *Thoracic Surgery Clinics* (part one was published in November 2007, Volume 17, Number 4) on thoracic anatomy provide not only a complete and in-depth revision of normal anatomy but also clinically and radiologically oriented concepts of traditional anatomy. As shown throughout both issues, the essential facts of anatomy found in early texts are still important, but they have evolved and developed into a more refined science that must be well known if one is to ensure that each patient gets the best possible operation for his or her thoracic disorder.

The creation of anatomy articles such as those can be achieved only through the assistance of numerous particularly creative and dedicated people. In this respect, we were privileged to be associated with Alex and David Baker of DNA Illustrations, Inc, who provided anatomically precise artwork and who understood the significant advances in electronic communication of anatomical details that have taken place over the past few years. Only a surgeon can appreciate the degree of patience and work involved in the making of such outstanding color sketches, which should be useful not only to students of thoracic surgery but also to practicing surgeons. The Bakers have taken great care to precisely correlate each author's thoughts with their own work in a scientific,

Thorac Surg Clin 21 (2011) xiii–xiv
doi:10.1016/j.thorsurg.2011.01.008
1547-4127/11/$ – see front matter © 2011 Elsevier Inc. All rights reserved.

enthusiastic, and professional manner. The process began with reference material taken from existing illustrations, photographs, operating room photographs, or even hand-drawn sketches scribbled on napkins. Based on these ideas, line drawings were made and they were sent to me and to individual authors for mutual review. After corrections had been made, color processing and scanning were done, and proofs of these color illustrations were sent again to me and to each author for final approval before being released to the publisher. Most importantly, the drawings were done in a homogeneous fashion throughout the books.

The hiring of expert medical artists able to create such impressive artwork would not have been possible without adequate financial support. We were thus very fortunate to have Johnson & Johnson Medical Products (Ethicon Canada) as our partners, and they provided the necessary funding for the anatomical illustrations. Without their dedicated support and commitment to academic excellence, it is obvious that we would never have been able to produce such work.

I am grateful to Doctor Mark Ferguson, Consulting Editor, and to Elsevier, for their open minds on the idea of publishing an atlas of thoracic anatomy. I would also like to personally thank and commend Catherine Bewick and Ruth Malwitz whose gracious acceptance of delays in production made my life a lot easier over the past few years. Finally, Marie-Hélène Lavoie, my administrative assistant has been a great and dependable help over the past few years, which has facilitated my work in many respects.

Jean Deslauriers, MD, FRCS(C)
Institut Universitaire de Cardiologie et de
Pneumologie de Québec
Laval University, 2725 Chemin Sainte-Foy
Quebec City, Quebec G1V 4G5, Canada

E-mail address:
jean.deslauriers@chg.ulaval.ca

Surface Anatomy and Surface Landmarks for Thoracic Surgery: Part II

Shona E. Smith, MD, FRCSC, Gail E. Darling, MD, FRCSC*

KEYWORDS

- Surface anatomy • Heart • Lungs • Pleura • Mediastinum
- Diaphragm

A thorough understanding of the surface anatomy is important to thoracic surgical trainees and surgeons alike, which involves studying not only the relationship of surface landmarks to their deeper structures but also how these landmarks are influenced by variability in patient body habitus, position, phase of respiration, and pathology. This knowledge enhances diagnostic and clinical examination skills as well as contributes to accurate interpretation of imaging of benign, traumatic, and malignant thoracic conditions. The knowledge of surface anatomy also facilitates safe completion of bedside procedures, including central venous access, thoracentesis, chest tube insertion, and pericardiocentesis. By studying the configuration of body surfaces and appreciating their relation to underlying structures, accurate thoracic incisions can be made that avoid the technical difficulties and complications arising from inadequate exposure. Surface projections of interest to the thoracic surgeon that are reviewed include those that define the location of the heart, great vessels, pleura, mediastinal structures, and diaphragm. Surface anatomy of the chest wall, including muscular and skeletal landmarks and pulmonary fissures, is not covered because it is covered in detail in an article by Sayeed and Darling elsewhere in this issue.

SURFACE ANATOMY OF THE TRACHEA, LUNGS, AND PLEURAE

Knowledge of the surface anatomy of the major airways, lungs, and pleurae is critical to localize pathology identified on imaging and clinical examination.

Trachea

The trachea, measuring 15 cm, begins at the lower border of the cricoid cartilage at the level of the sixth cervical vertebra. With the head in neutral position, its proximal 5 cm can be palpated just superior to the suprasternal notch, which is in line with the second thoracic vertebra. With the neck extended, as in preparation for a tracheotomy, up to 8 cm of the trachea is palpable. The trachea descends vertically to enter the thorax behind the manubrium just right of midline and bifurcates at the carina at the level of the sternal angle (**Fig. 1**). This bifurcation corresponds to the level of the lower border of the fourth thoracic vertebra. The surface projection of the carina can move 2 to 3 cm with respiration to reach the level of the fifth or sixth thoracic vertebra.

Major Airways

The trachea ends at the carina, where it divides into the right and left main stem bronchi. The right main stem bronchus travels 2.5 cm downwards at 25° from vertical before entering the right lung hilum at the level of the fifth thoracic vertebral body. The left main stem bronchus travels 5 cm in a less vertical trajectory, approximately 45° from vertical. The left main stem bronchus meets the left lung hilum at the level of the sixth thoracic vertebra.

Division of Thoracic Surgery, Toronto General Hospital, University of Toronto, 200 Elizabeth Street, 9N955, Toronto, Ontario M5G 2C4, Canada
* Corresponding author.
E-mail address: gail.darling@uhn.on.ca

Thorac Surg Clin 21 (2011) 139–155
doi:10.1016/j.thorsurg.2011.01.004
1547-4127/11/$ – see front matter © 2011 Elsevier Inc. All rights reserved.

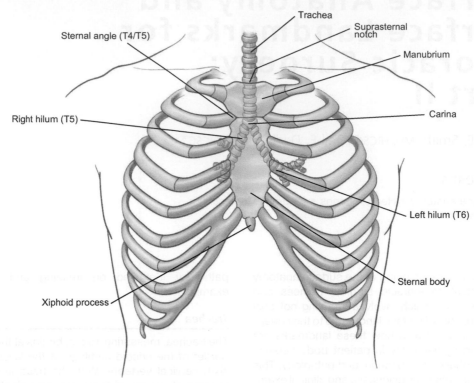

Fig. 1. Surface relations of the trachea and major airways.

The hila of the lung lie posterior to the second to fourth costal cartilages, 2.5 cm lateral to the sternal edge or 5 cm from the spinous processes of the fourth to sixth vertebra when approached from the back.

Pleura

The reflection of the parietal pleura, following the contour of the thoracic cavity, reflects the limits of lung expansion. The cervical pleura follows a line from the medial third of the clavicle upward to extend 2.5 cm above the clavicle The upper border of the pleura called the cupola or dome lies behind the sternocleidomastoid muscle, 2 cm below the cricoid cartilage. The line of the pleura then extends inferiorly toward the sterno-clavicular joint and then to the midline at the sternal angle. It continues midline along the sternum to the level of the fourth costal cartilage. Here the pleura diverges. On the right side, the parietal pleura continues inferiorly to the right of the xiphisternal joint. On the left, the pleura is deflected laterally starting at the level of the fourth costal cartilage to reach the left lateral aspect of the sternum by the sixth costal cartilage. The pleura then continues along the left margin of the sternum to the xiphisternal joint. Inferiorly, the parietal pleura extends beyond the lung to cover the diaphragm, resulting in a true space between the parietal pleura and the lung covered by visceral pleura. Areas of separation are defined as the costodiaphragmatic recess and the costomediastinal recess (**Figs. 2** and **3**). The costodiaphragmatic recess reaches the level of the neck of the 12th rib on each side of the vertebrae. In this area, with expiration, the lung lies approximately 5 cm (or 2 rib spaces) higher than the parietal pleural reflection. This area can increase to a distance as far as 7.5 cm with deep respiration. Anteriorly, the left parietal pleura follows the diaphragm under the left lower costal cartilages to extend into the retrosternal costomediastinal recess. Laterally, the pleura follows the contour of the ribs, crossing the eighth rib in the midclavicular line, the tenth rib in the midaxillary line, and the twelfth rib at the lateral border of the erector spinae.

Lungs

In healthy individuals, at the apical dome and cost-overtebral border, the lung and its adherent visceral pleura are separated from the parietal

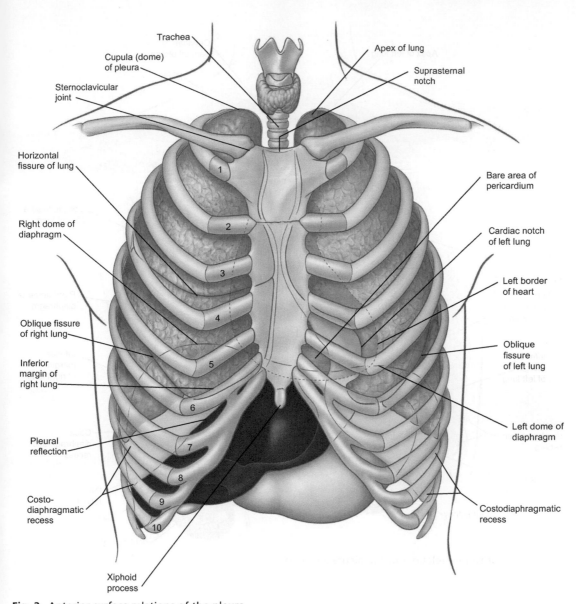

Trachea

Cupula (dome)
of pleura

Sternoclavicular
joint

Apex of lung

Suprasternal
notch

Horizontal
fissure of lung

1

Bare area of
pericardium

Right dome of
diaphragm

2

Cardiac notch
of left lung

3

Left border
of heart

4

Oblique fissure
of right lung

Oblique
fissure
of left lung

Inferior
margin of
right lung

5

6

Pleural
reflection

7

Left dome of
diaphragm

8

Costo-
diaphragmatic
recess

9

10

Costodiaphragmatic
recess

Xiphoid
process

Fig. 2. Anterior surface relations of the pleura.

pleura only by a thin film of pleural fluid. Therefore, the surface markings of the lung are nearly identical to those of the pleurae. The apex of the lung, lying 2.5 cm above the medial third of the clavicle anteriorly, puts it at risk of puncture and subsequent pneumothorax with insertion of internal jugular or subclavian central venous line catheters. Posteriorly, the apex comes as high as the 7th cervical vertebra, 5 cm from midline. From there, the surface projection of the lungs descends posteriorly on either side of the vertebral column down to the level of the 10th thoracic vertebra (see **Fig. 3**). Anteriorly, the lung follows the parietal pleura from the apex inferiorly to the sternoclavicular joint and then to the midline at the sternal angle. The lung continues in the midline to the level of the fourth costal cartilage and then deflects laterally such that the inferior border on the right crosses the midclavicular line at the level of sixth rib and reaches the level of eighth rib at the midaxillary line (see **Fig. 2**; **Fig. 4**). On the left, the lung breaks from the pleura at the cardiac notch and curves away from the midline to lie 2.5 cm from the pleura and sternum at the level of the fifth costal cartilage and 4 cm from the midline at the level of the sixth costal cartilage. Similar to the

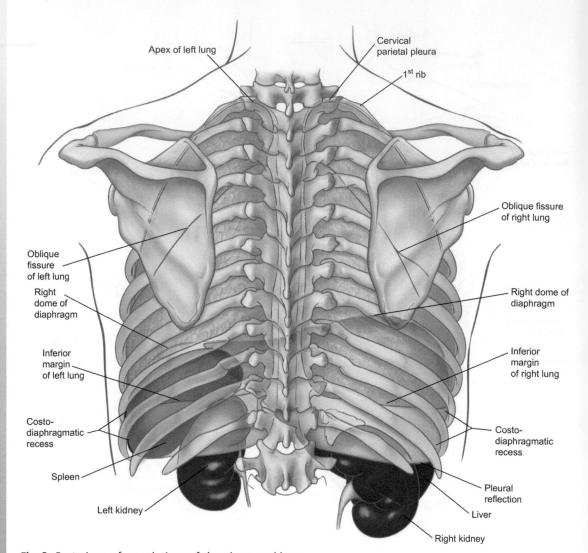

Apex of left lung

Cervical
parietal pleura

1ˢᵗ rib

Oblique fissure
of right lung

Oblique
fissure
of left lung

Right
dome of
diaphragm

Right dome of
diaphragm

Inferior
margin
of left lung

Inferior
margin
of right lung

Costo-
diaphragmatic
recess

Costo-
diaphragmatic
recess

Spleen

Pleural
reflection

Left kidney

Liver

Right kidney

Fig. 3. Posterior surface relations of the pleura and lung.

right lung, the inferior aspect of the left lung crosses the midclavicular line at the level of the sixth rib and the midaxillary line at the level of the eighth rib. With full inspiration, the lung moves down 5 to 8 cm.

Pulmonary Fissures

The fissures of the lung, dividing the right lung into 3 lobes and the left lung into 2 lobes, can also be identified by surface projections. The oblique fissure of the right lung approximately follows the line of the fifth rib, starting at the fourth thoracic spinous process and ending near the sixth costochondral junction (see **Figs. 2** and **3**). The position of the oblique fissure of the left lung is more

variable. The left oblique fissure generally follows a line from the third or fourth thoracic vertebra curving around to the sixth costochondral junction, crossing the midaxillary line at the fifth rib. Both fissures move down 2 to 5 cm with inspiration and may be incomplete or may extend as far as the lung hilum. With patients' arms raised above their shoulders, the oblique fissure approximates the line of the medial border of their scapula. On the right, between the upper and middle lobes, the horizontal (transverse) fissure extends on a line from the right fourth costal cartilage at the anterior border of the lung to the oblique fissure approximately at the fifth intercostal space in the midaxillary line (see **Fig. 4**). The right middle lobe is therefore located as a triangle between the right

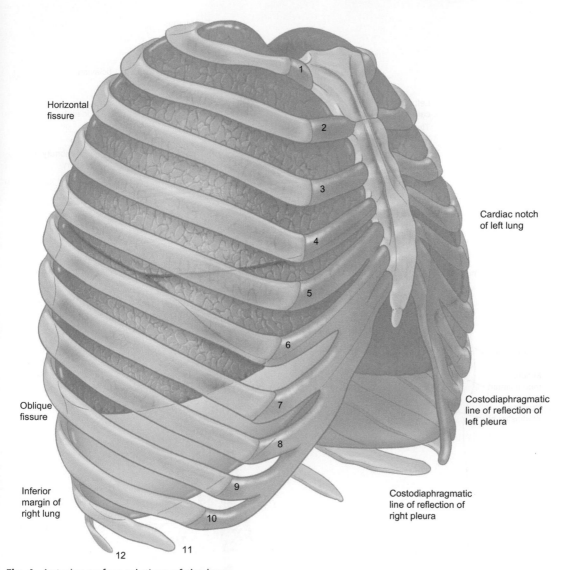

Horizontal fissure

Cardiac notch of left lung

Oblique fissure

Costodiaphragmatic line of reflection of left pleura

Inferior margin of right lung

Costodiaphragmatic line of reflection of right pleura

1 2 3 4 5 6 7 8 9 10 11 12

Fig. 4. Anterior surface relations of the lung.

fourth rib at the sternal edge, fifth rib at the midaxillary line, and the sixth rib at the midclavicular line (see **Fig. 4**). The upper and middle lobes are anterior to the oblique fissure, whereas the lower lobes lie posteriorly.

SURFACE ANATOMY OF THE MEDIASTINUM

The mediastinum, defined as the area between the lungs, is bordered by the thoracic vertebral column posteriorly and the sternum anteriorly. The mediastinum is traditionally divided into 2 parts: superior and inferior. The inferior mediastinum is further compartmentalized into anterior, middle, and posterior portions (**Fig. 5**). The superior mediastinum lies below the line of the first rib, which is often referred

to as the plane of the thoracic inlet. It is separated form the inferior mediastinum by the sternal plane formed by a line joining the sternomanubrial joint to the inferior surface of the fourth thoracic vertebra. The superior mediastinum lies between the manubrium, upper 4 thoracic vertebrae, and mediastinal pleura. Important superior mediastinal structures include the great vessels, vagus, phrenic and left recurrent laryngeal nerves, trachea, esophagus, thoracic duct, and lymph nodes.

The anterior mediastinum contains lymph nodes and thymic gland remnants and is bounded by the pericardium and sternum (see **Fig. 5**). The posterior mediastinum contains the vagus and splanchnic nerves, esophagus, thoracic duct, lymph nodes, as well as the descending thoracic

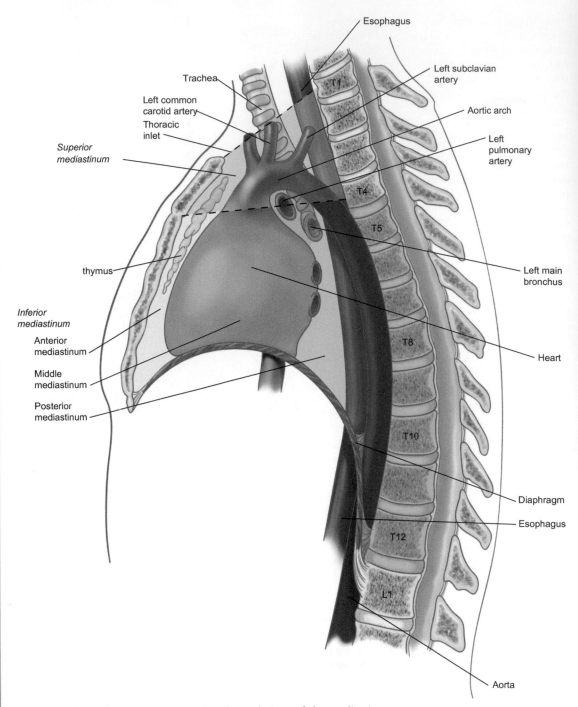

Fig. 5. Mediastinal compartments and surface relations of the mediastinum.

aorta and azygos and hemiazygos veins. The posterior mediastinum is situated between the 4th to 12th thoracic vertebrae and the mediastinal pleura (see **Fig. 5**).

The middle mediastinum with the heart, pericardium, carina, main bronchi, pulmonary vessels, phrenic nerves, cardiac plexus, and lymph nodes lies in between the anterior and posterior parts (see **Fig. 5**).

Heart

The heart and pericardium are located in the middle mediastinum, with two-thirds of the heart's mass to the left of midline. The heart is bounded by the sternum and costal cartilages of the third to sixth ribs anteriorly; lungs laterally; and pulmonary hila, carina, bronchi, and esophagus posteriorly (**Fig. 6**). When lying supine as for a sternotomy, the atria are found to the right of the ventricles, and the right atrium and ventricle are anterior to the left atrium and ventricle. The right lung extending over the midline overlaps the side of the heart. On the left, the lung extends only to the level of the cardiac notch at the fourth costal cartilage and does not cross the midline (see **Fig. 2**). The heart is encased by 2 layers of pericardium: the inner visceral pericardium that lies in direct contact with the heart and attaches to the great vessels and diaphragm and the outer parietal pericardium that forms the inner layer of the pericardial sac. The pericardium has the same surface projections as the heart, except that its right border extends more superiorly to the level of the second cartilage to wrap around the superior vena cava.

The long axis of the heart lies along a line between the left epigastrium and right shoulder, parallel to the interventricular septum separating the left and right sides of the heart. The short axis corresponds to the atrioventricular groove or coronary sinus, which separates the atrial and ventricular areas. The short axis is oriented obliquely, perpendicular to the long axis from the left third to the right sixth sternal ends of the costal cartilages (see **Fig. 6**). The surface projections of the sternocostal surface of the heart can be visualized as a trapezoid connected between 4 points (**Fig. 7**). The right heart border is formed by the right atrium and can be drawn as a convex line from a point just lateral to the sternum at the superior border of the right third costal cartilage (A) to the right sixth or seventh costochondral junction approximately 1 to 2 cm lateral to the sternal edge (B). Continuing this line superiorly reveals the border of the superior vena cava; inferiorly this line outlines the border of the inferior vena cava. Extending a line from point (B) to the

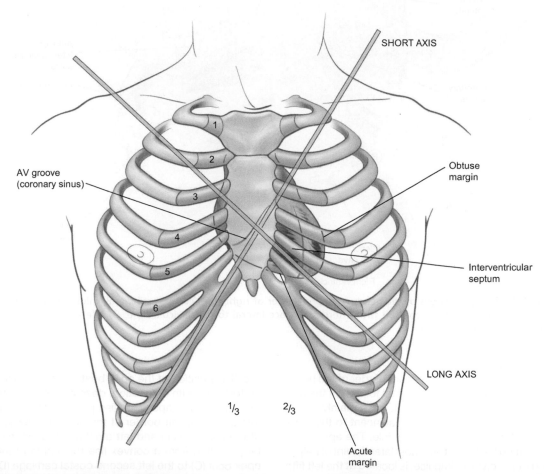

Fig. 6. Surface projections of the heart atrioventricular groove and interventricular septum. AV, atrioventricular.

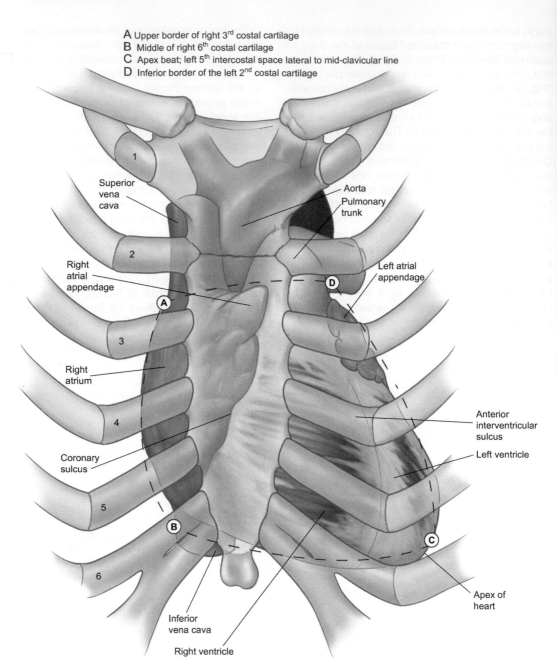

A Upper border of right 3rd costal cartilage
B Middle of right 6th costal cartilage
C Apex beat; left 5th intercostal space lateral to mid-clavicular line
D Inferior border of the left 2nd costal cartilage

Fig. 7. Surface projections of the heart. A, upper border of right third costal cartilage; B, middle of right sixth costal cartilage; C, apex beat, left fifth intercostal space lateral to midclavicular line; D, inferior border of the left second costal cartilage.

apex beat (C) draws the inferior border of the heart. Reaching the level of the central tendon of the diaphragm, this lower border is formed mainly by the right ventricle except 1.5 cm adjacent to the apex that is formed by the left ventricle. The apex beat, indicating the lowest and most lateral point of palpation of the cardiac impulse, is located at the left fifth intercostal space just medial to the midclavicular line. The position of the apex beat, which can vary up to 10 cm with respiration, does not correlate to the true cardiac apex that lies just inferolateral to this point. The left border of the heart, composed of the left ventricle and left atrial appendage, can bo projected from a convex line running from the apex beat (C) to the left second costal cartilage (D) approximately 1 cm from the left sternal edge. The superior border runs from (A) to (D) and is composed of the 2 atria. Considered the base of the heart, the superior border is where the major systemic and pulmonic vessels originate.

The surface projections of the valves lie in close proximity to the atrioventricular groove (see **Fig. 6**; **Fig. 8**). The pulmonary valve lies partially behind the superior border of the left third costal cartilage and partially behind the left sternum as a 2.5-cm horizontal line. The pulmonary trunk lies parallel to this line at the level of the left second costal cartilage. The aortic valve lies inferior and to the right of the pulmonary valve. The orifice of the aortic valve is 2.5 cm long, extending from the medial end of the

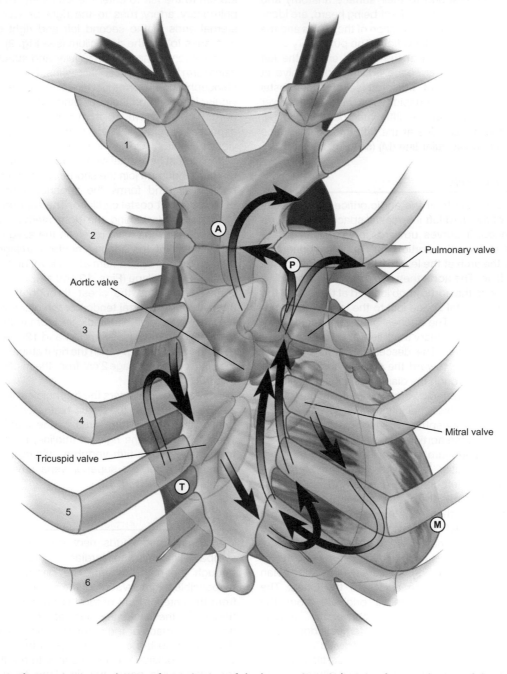

Fig. 8. Surface projection and areas of auscultation of the heart valves. A, location for auscultation of the aortic valve; P, location for aucultation of the pulmonary valve; T, location for auscultation of the tricuspid valve; M, location for auscultation of the mitral valve.

left third intercostal space down and to the right. The tricuspid orifice, 4 cm long, starts just below the level of the fourth right costal cartilage, descending to the right to the level of the fifth costal cartilage. The mitral orifice, measuring 3 cm, starts behind the sternum at the level of the left fourth costal cartilage and passes down and to the right.

The areas of auscultation for the cardiac valves do not correspond to their surface anatomy and instead, depending on best being heard, are identified based on the orientation of the valves and the direction of their blood flow. The pulmonary valve is best auscultated at the sternal end of the left second intercostal space (P), the aortic valve at the sternal end of the right second intercostal space (A), the tricuspid valve at the left lower sternal border at the fifth intercostal space (T), and the mitral valve at the fifth intercostal space at the midclavicular line (M) (see **Fig. 8**).

Great Vessels

The aorta starts at the aortic orifice at the medial end of the third left intercostal space. As the aorta ascends, it curves upward, forward, and to the right to form the aortic arch. The manubrium lies over the arch at the level of the second right costal cartilage. The aorta then becomes the descending aorta with the aortic knob located at the level of the first intercostal space just to the left of the manubrium (**Fig. 9**). The tracheal bifurcation (at the level of T4) and pulmonary trunk lie within the shadow of the aortic arch. The descending aorta continues down moving toward the midline and enters the abdomen through the diaphragmatic aortic hiatus, at the 12th thoracic vertebra, approximately 9 cm below the xiphisternal junction (**Figs. 10–12**).

The brachiocephalic or innominate artery originates from the aortic arch at a point at the middle of the manubrium and then ascends to the right sternoclavicular joint where it bifurcates (see **Fig. 9**). The left common carotid artery arises just left to the middle of the manubrium before it ascends to the left sternoclavicular joint (see **Fig. 9**). The left subclavian artery arises from the aortic arch behind the left border of the manubrium and also ascends to behind the left sternoclavicular joint (see **Fig. 9**). Bilaterally, the subclavian arteries run over the apices of the lungs. The internal mammary arteries originate from the subclavian arteries 2 cm above the clavicle between the heads of the sternocleidomastoid muscle. Bilaterally each artery travels down and medially toward the second costal cartilage before reaching the sixth cartilage where it bifurcates into the superior epigastric and musculophrenic arteries. These arteries lie 1 to 2 cm lateral to the

sternal border, deep to the costal cartilages and internal intercostal muscles.

The pulmonary trunk is 2.5 cm wide and 5 cm long. The trunk originates from the pulmonary orifice at the third left chondrosternal joint. The vessel runs up to the left to the level of its bifurcation at the second left costal cartilage, 1 cm from the sternal edge. The left pulmonary artery runs 2.5 cm to the left to enter the left hilum. The right pulmonary artery runs to the right between the sternal ends of the second left and right costal cartilages to join the right hilum (see **Fig. 9**).

The union of the internal jugular and subclavian veins form the brachiocephalic veins. The right brachiocephalic vein forms just lateral to the sternoclavicular junction and then descends along the right border of the sternum, from behind the medial aspect of the clavicle lateral to the right sternoclavicular junction. On the left, the brachiocephalic vein is almost horizontal where it crosses the superior manubrium to join the shorter right brachiocephalic vein and forms the superior vena cava behind the first costal cartilage. The superior vena cava descends behind the right sternal border. The superior vena cava receives the azygos vein at the level of the second costal cartilage and then enters the right atrium at the level of the third right costal cartilage (**Figs. 13 and 14**). The inferior vena cava enters the chest through the caval opening of the central tendon of the diaphragm at the level of the eighth thoracic vertebra to the right of the xiphisternum (see **Figs. 11 and 12**). The inferior vena cava runs up to join the right atrium behind the sixth costal cartilage 2 cm from the midline (see **Fig. 13**).

The azygos vein enters the thoracic cavity either beside the aorta at the aortic hiatus or independently through the right crus of the diaphragm. The vein runs to the right of midline, running up to the level of the fifth vertebra, where it arches forward to enter the superior vena cava at the sternal angle (see **Fig. 13**).

Nerves

The phrenic and vagus nerves as well as the sympathetic trunk and cardiac plexus all course through the mediastinum. The phrenic nerves, responsible for innervation of the diaphragm, arise from the anterior rami of the third to fifth cervical nerves. In the neck, the phrenic nerves course along the surface of the anterior scalene muscles descending to the clavicle between the 2 heads of the sternocleidomastoid muscle. In the thorax, the left phrenic nerve travels along the medial surface of the left pleura following a line from the sternal end of the left clavicle to the left lateral

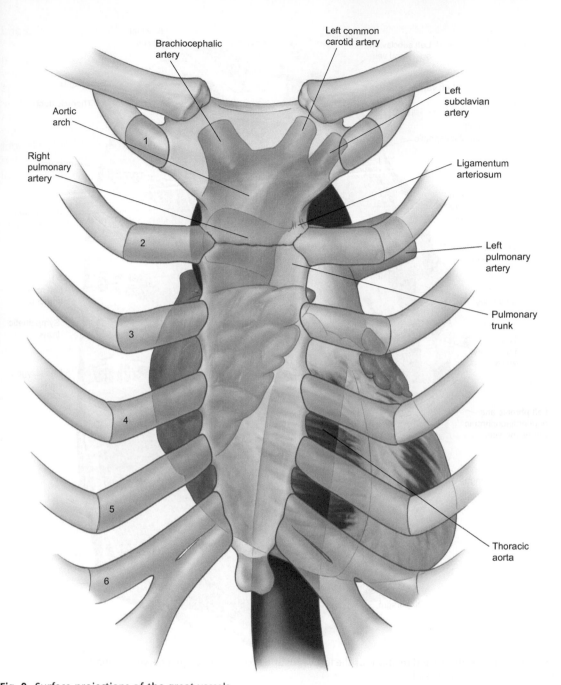

Fig. 9. Surface projections of the great vessels.

aspect of the manubrium at the first intercostals space and finally along the left border of the heart. The right phrenic nerve follows the medial surface of the right pleura following a line along the right side of the right brachiocephalic vein, the superior vena cava, the right border of the heart, and the inferior vena cava. The surface markings of these structures are described earlier. Both phrenic nerves pass posterior to the internal mammary arteries bilaterally and then descend anterior to the pulmonary hilum along the heart borders in between the pericardium and mediastinal pleura before branching out onto the diaphragm (see **Figs. 10** and **14**).

The paired vagus nerves, providing cholinergic, efferent, and afferent fibers, enter the thorax posterior to the phrenic nerves running beside the common carotid arteries and trachea (see **Figs. 10** and **14**). The right vagus nerve gives off a recurrent laryngeal branch that passes around

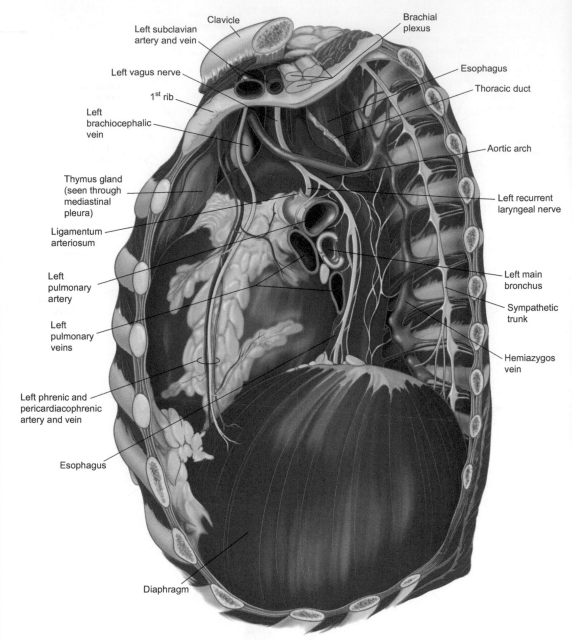

Fig. 10. Left hemithorax and relations of the left vagus and recurrent laryngeal nerves, sympathetic chain, pulmonary hilum, and great vessels.

the right subclavian artery before ascending back to the neck in the tracheoesophageal groove. The left recurrent laryngeal nerve branches off the left vagus nerve after it crosses over the aortic arch. The laryngeal nerve loops around the aorta just lateral to the ligamentum arteriosum at the fourth thoracic vertebra to ascend to the neck (see **Fig. 10**). Both vagi nerve course posterior to the pulmonary hilum sending branches to the pulmonary and then esophageal plexuses and

then exit the thorax with the esophagus at the level of the tenth thoracic vertebra (see **Fig. 10**).

The sympathetic trunk runs down from the neck through the thorax to the abdomen just lateral to the vertebral column (see **Fig. 10**). The trunk passes over the head of the ribs and behind the medial arcuate ligament. The cardiac plexus, formed by bilateral branches from the cervical sympathetic trunks, vagi nerves, and recurrent nerves, sends branches to the lungs and heart (see **Fig. 10**).

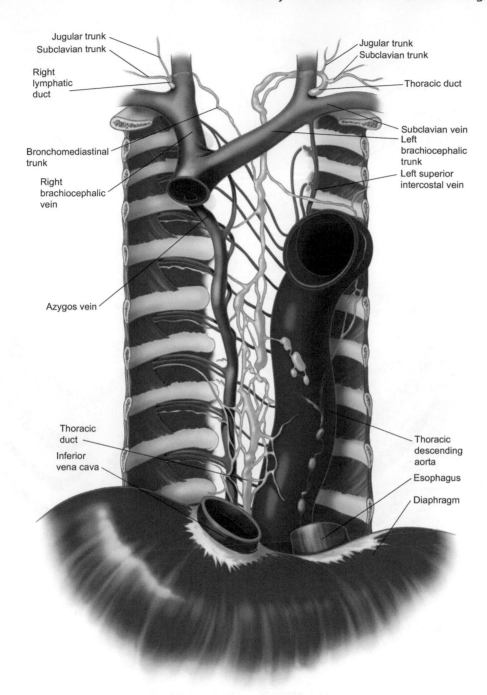

Jugular trunk
Subclavian trunk
Right lymphatic duct
Bronchomediastinal trunk
Right brachiocephalic vein
Azygos vein
Thoracic duct
Inferior vena cava

Jugular trunk
Subclavian trunk
Thoracic duct
Subclavian vein
Left brachiocephalic trunk
Left superior intercostal vein
Thoracic descending aorta
Esophagus
Diaphragm

Fig. 11. Relations of the thoracic duct.

Thoracic Duct

The thoracic duct starts in the abdomen at the confluence of lymphatic trunks or cisterna chyli to the right of midline at the level of the lower border of the 12th vertebral body 10 cm below the xiphisternal joint. The thoracic duct runs up in the posterior midline anterior to the lower eighth thoracic vertebrae between the azygos vein and descending thoracic aorta (see **Fig. 11**). The thoracic duct enters the thoracic cavity through the aortic hiatus of the diaphragm at the 12th thoracic vertebra (see **Fig. 12**). Crossing to the left approximately at the level of the fifth thoracic

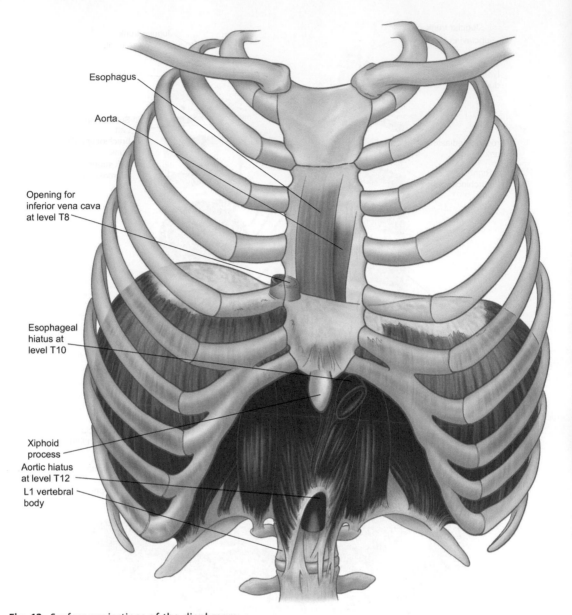

Esophagus

Aorta

Opening for
inferior vena cava
at level T8

Esophageal
hiatus at
level T10

Xiphoid
process

Aortic hiatus
at level T12

L1 vertebral
body

Fig. 12. Surface projections of the diaphragm.

vertebral body, the thoracic duct then ascends into the superior mediastinum to the left side of the esophagus, running behind the aortic arch and left subclavian artery until reaching the thoracic inlet. As the thoracic duct enters the neck, it arches at the level of the transverse process of the seventh cervical vertebra, up to 4 cm above the clavicle, where it is susceptible to damage during insertion of left internal jugular central lines. The thoracic duct courses posterior to the carotid sheath and then downwards in front of the cervical portion of the left subclavian artery to insert into the junction of the left subclavian and internal jugular veins (see **Fig. 11**).

SURFACE PROJECTION OF THE DIAPHRAGM

The diaphragm separates the thoracic from the abdominal cavity. The diaphragm is convex toward the thorax, concave toward the abdomen, high anteriorly, and low posteriorly. The position of the apex of the diaphragm is strongly influenced by body habitus, position, respiration, and intra-thoracic and intra-abdominal pathology. The right

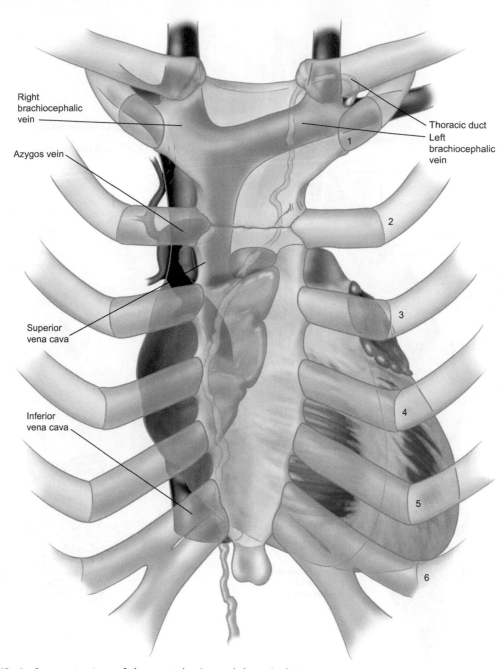

Right brachiocephalic vein

Azygos vein

Superior vena cava

Inferior vena cava

Thoracic duct

Left brachiocephalic vein

1

2

3

4

5

6

Fig. 13. Surface projections of the central veins and thoracic duct.

hemidiaphragm with forced expiration rises to the level of the fourth costal cartilage and to the fifth on the left. With full inspiration, the diaphragm descends on the right to the sixth rib or tenth thoracic vertebra. The left rises approximately 1 cm less. The central tendon lies at level with the xiphisternal junction.

The muscular attachments of the diaphragm account for its shape. The costal portion attaches

low to the internal surfaces of the lower 6 costal cartilages and their ribs. The lumbar portion originates from the medial and lateral arcuate ligaments, transversus abdominis, and third and fourth lumbar vertebra. The sternal portion attaches high. At the level of the costodiaphragmatic recess, the lung overlaps the intra-abdominal viscera located below the dome of the diaphragm: the liver, stomach, and spleen. Also,

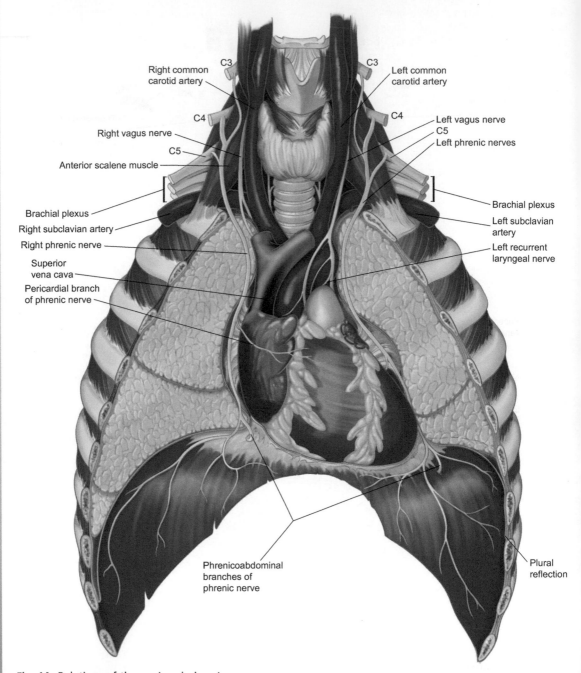

Right common carotid artery — C3

C3 — Left common carotid artery

C4

Right vagus nerve

C5

Anterior scalene muscle

C4

Left vagus nerve
C5
Left phrenic nerves

Brachial plexus

Right subclavian artery

Right phrenic nerve

Superior vena cava

Pericardial branch of phrenic nerve

Brachial plexus

Left subclavian artery

Left recurrent laryngeal nerve

Phrenicoabdominal branches of phrenic nerve

Plural reflection

Fig. 14. Relations of the vagi and phrenic nerves.

the heart lies above and anterior to the gastric fundus with some overlap (**Fig. 14**). The overlap is important to consider in evaluating penetrating wounds of the thorax or abdomen.

The diaphragm allows passage of several important structures between the thorax and abdomen (see **Fig. 12**). The inferior vena cava and right phrenic nerve pass through the central tendon of the diaphragm 2.5 cm to the right of

the midline at the level of the eighth thoracic vertebra, behind the right sixth costal cartilage. The esophagus, anterior and posterior vagal trunks, and esophageal branches of the left gastric artery all pass through the esophageal hiatus, which is located 2.5 cm left of midline and is composed of a sling of fibers from the right crus at the level of the tenth thoracic vertebra, behind the left seventh costal cartilage. The aortic hiatus lies to the left of the midline behind the median arcuate ligament of the diaphragm, at level with the body of the 12th thoracic vertebra. The aortic hiatus allows passage of the descending aorta, thoracic duct, and azygos vein. The azygos vein may also pass through an opening lateral to or through the right crus of the diaphragm.

SUMMARY

Surface anatomy is an integral part of a thoracic surgeon's armamentarium to assist with the diagnosis, staging, and treatment of thoracic pathology. As reviewed in this article, the surface landmarks of the lungs, heart, great vessels, and mediastinum are critical for appropriate patient care and should be learned in conjunction with classic anatomy.

FURTHER READINGS

Basmajian JV. Surface anatomy: an instruction manual. 2nd edition. Baltimore (MD): Williams & Wilkins; 1983.

Gray HS, Standring S. Gray's anatomy: the anatomical basis of clinical practice. 39th edition. Edinburgh (UK): Elsevier Churchill Livingstone; 2005.

Keogh B, Ebbs S. Normal surface anatomy. London: William Heinemann Medical Books Limited; 1984.

Lumley JSP. Surface anatomy: the anatomical basis of clinical examination. 3rd edition. Edinburgh (UK): Churchill Livingstone, Imprint of Elsevier Limited; 2002.

Pearson FG. Thoracic surgery. 2nd edition. New York: Churchill Livingstone; 2002.

Robinson A, Jamieson EB. Surface anatomy. London: Humphrey Milford Oxford Medical Publications; 1928.

Sayeed RA, Darling GE. Surface anatomy and surface landmarks for thoracic surgery. Thorac Surg Clin 2007;17(4):449–61.

Waterson D. Anatomy in the living model: a handbook for the study of the surface, movements, and mechanics of the human body and for the surface projection of the viscera, etc. London: Hodder and Stoughton Limited; 1931.

Anatomy of the Pleura

David J. Finley, MD*, Valerie W. Rusch, MD

KEYWORDS

- Pleural anatomy • Stomata • Visceral • Parietal
- Lymphatics

During development, to protect vital organs, the thoracic cavity is formed to house the lungs, heart, and mediastinal structures. This rigid encasement shields these organs from injury, but inhibits their ability to move freely. The pleura allows the lung to expand and contract within this space, and also transmits the mechanical forces of the diaphragm and chest wall with minimal friction and damage to the lung parenchyma and protects the lung from infection. The anatomy of the pleural space provides insight into how this complex layer performs all of these functions.

GROSS ANATOMY

The pleural space is defined by the visceral and parietal pleura, and contains a small amount of liquid to help facilitate the expansion and contraction of the lung and chest wall.[1] The visceral pleura covers the lung from the pulmonary hilum outward and lines all of the major and minor fissures, including two opposing layers that form the inferior pulmonary ligament (triangular ligament) (**Fig. 1**). The inferior pulmonary ligament is created through invagination of the lung as it grows into the thoracic cavity, pulling along the ventral and dorsal aspects of the visceral pleura (**Fig. 2**).[2] Because no defined plane exists between the lung and the visceral pleura, which is densely adherent to the elastic layer of the lung, its removal can cause tearing of the underlying lung parenchyma.[3]

The extension of the pleura into the interlobar spaces allow for each individual lobe to expand and contract separately.[2] If one lobe has an abnormality, such as occlusion of a segmental bronchus by tumor or secretions, the other ipsilateral lobes are often not restricted by its collapse. In many people these separations of the lobes, or fissures, by the visceral pleura are incomplete or septated, reducing the ability of the lung to tolerate these insults to one lobe.

The inner surface of the chest wall, mediastinum, and diaphragm are covered by the parietal pleura, and the transition between the parietal and visceral pleura is at the level of the pulmonary hilum.[4] A fat plane between the parietal pleura and the endothoracic fascia is present along most of the chest wall, allowing the pleura to be removed easily from the basilar structures. This plane is often lost through fusion of the parietal pleura to the underlying structures, especially along the pericardium and diaphragm, making the parietal pleura over these areas difficult to remove.

Within the thoracic cavity, the pleura extends 2 to 3 cm superiorly above the first rib, rising up beneath the sternocleidomastoid muscle, forming the cupola, or dome of the lung (**Fig. 3**). The inferior aspect of the pleural space varies from anterior to lateral to posterior, following the line of attachment between the diaphragm and the chest wall. Anteriorly, the pleura ends at the level of the sixth or seventh rib and, coursing at an oblique angle, it can reach below the twelfth rib posteriorly (**Fig. 4**).[5] Because the pleura stretches beyond the confines of the rib cage, injury in these areas is more common during procedures, increasing risk of pneumothorax.

Thoracic Service, Department of Surgery, Memorial Sloan-Kettering Cancer Center, 1275 York Avenue, New York, NY 10065, USA
* Corresponding author.
E-mail address: finleyd1@mskcc.org

Thorac Surg Clin 21 (2011) 157–163
doi:10.1016/j.thorsurg.2010.12.001
1547-4127/11/$ – see front matter © 2011 Published by Elsevier Inc.

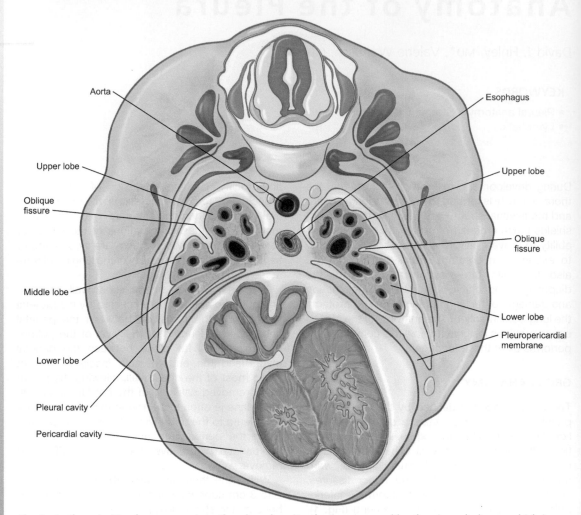

Fig. 1. As the primitive lungs grow into the pleural cavity, they are covered by the visceral pleura, which invaginates with the lung buds.

The visceral and parietal pleura are serosal membranes, but only the parietal pleura is believed to contain stomata.[6,7] The parietal pleura becomes thick and strong at the level of the diaphragm. It also is attached to the multiple suspensory ligaments at the level of the diaphragmatic hiatus. The pleural sinuses are where the parietal pleura is in contact at the end of expiration and filled with lung during inspiration. They include the anterior and posterior costomediastinal sinuses, costophrenic sinus, and mediastinophrenic sinus.

EMBRYOLOGY

During the third week of gestation, the mesoderm differentiates to create the lateral mesoderm as one of the early precursors of the pleural sac. The lateral mesoderm forms the somatic and splanchnic mesoderms, which will become the parietal and visceral pleura, respectively.[4] The diaphragm then splits the somatic and splanchnic mesoderms to form the peritoneal and pleural sacs during the seventh week of gestation. The pleural cavity is complete within the third month, with the formation of lung buds that invaginate the visceral pleura over its surface (**Fig. 5**).

BLOOD SUPPLY

Some disagreement still exists on the blood supply to the visceral pleura. Originally, McLaughlin and colleagues[8,9] found that the visceral pleura was supplied by either the pulmonary artery or the bronchial artery. Evaluation of sheep visceral pleura showed exclusive supply

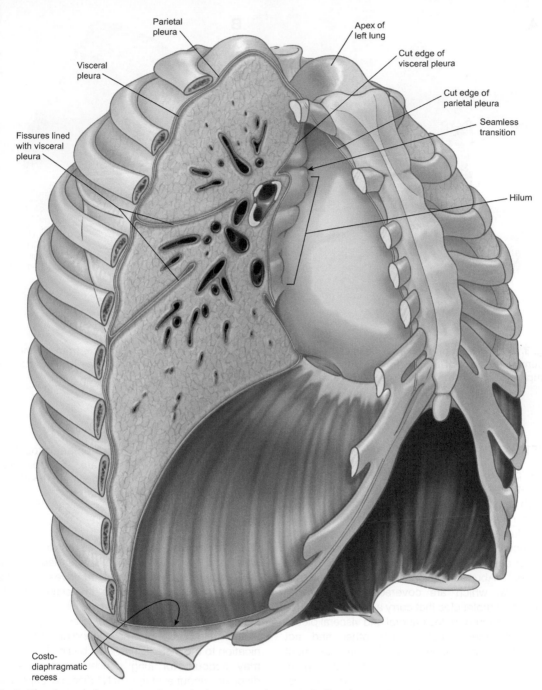

Parietal
pleura

Apex of
left lung

Cut edge of
visceral pleura

Cut edge of
parietal pleura

Seamless
transition

Visceral
pleura

Fissures lined
with visceral
pleura

Hilum

Costo-
diaphragmatic
recess

Fig. 2. The visceral pleura covers the entire lung parenchyma, including the intralobar fissures. There is a seamless transition to the parietal pleura at the level of the pulmonary hilum.

by the bronchial arteries.[10] Recent studies confirm that the pulmonary and systemic (bronchial) arterial systems feed the visceral pleura, but that the bronchial arteries are the main supply.[11] Venous return is through the pulmonary system. The parietal pleura arterial supply is from the systemic system, drawing on the arteries it covers (eg, the cupola parietal pleura derives its blood from the subclavian artery), with venous return in a similar fashion.

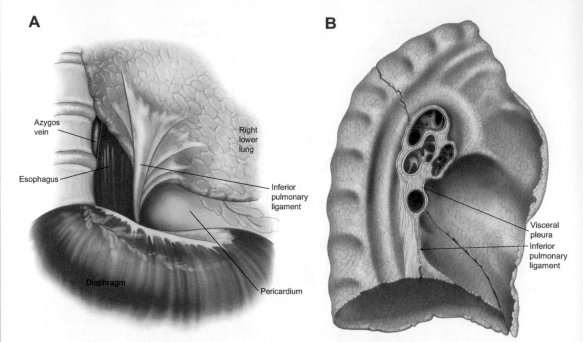

Fig. 3. (*A*) The inferior pulmonary ligament, also known as the triangular ligament, emanates from the mediastinum at the level of the junction of the esophagus and pericardium. (*B*) It tethers the lower lobe, containing lymphatic tissue and blood vessels sandwiched between two layers of visceral pleura.

HISTOLOGY

The pleura is composed of a monolayer of mesothelial cells layered over connective tissue. Much more complex than originally believed, these mesothelial cells have a rich endoplasmic reticulum (ER) and golgi complex that are believed to function for absorption and phagocytosis, playing an active role in the clearance of the pleural space.[3,4] Abundant microvilli line the surface of the cells, which are covered in oligolamellar surfactant molecules that carry a charge. Because they are layered on the parietal and visceral pleura microvilli, they repulse each other and act as graphite-like lubrication.[1,4] The basement membrane has a rich complex of elastic fibers, blood vessels, lymphatics, and nerve endings, allowing the cells to stretch with the underlying structures.

The visceral pleura is directly adherent to the elastic network of the lung, allowing distribution of the mechanical forces that are produced with inspiration, and transmission of the recoil forces to help expiration.[3,12,13] The rich network of lymphatics contained in the basement membrane helps to evacuate the fluid that accumulates within the periphery of the lung. In multiple animal species, including humans, the parietal pleura is more consistently found with stomata throughout its surface.[6,14–16] The stomata, or openings, provide direct communication between the pleural space and the lymphatics.

LYMPHATIC DRAINAGE

The rich network of lymphatics that runs through the basement membrane of the visceral pleura, especially within the lower lobes, removes fluid that has accumulated within the interstitium of the pulmonary parenchyma. These channels drain mainly to the intralobar and hilar lymph node stations. However, some have found direct communication to the mediastinal nodal basins,[15,17] which may account for lung cancers that have N2 disease without evidence of N1 disease, especially in the upper lobes. The visceral pleura plays a minor, if any, role in the clearance of pleural fluid or particles and does not seem to have direct communication to the lymphatics via stomata.

The parietal pleura contains several stomata, ranging from 2 to 12 μm in diameter.[4,14] These openings allow fluid to drain into the subpleural lymphatic system, mainly on the diaphragmatic, mediastinal, and inferior costal surfaces.[14] The lymphatic channels have endoluminal valves that facilitate movement of fluid and particles from the

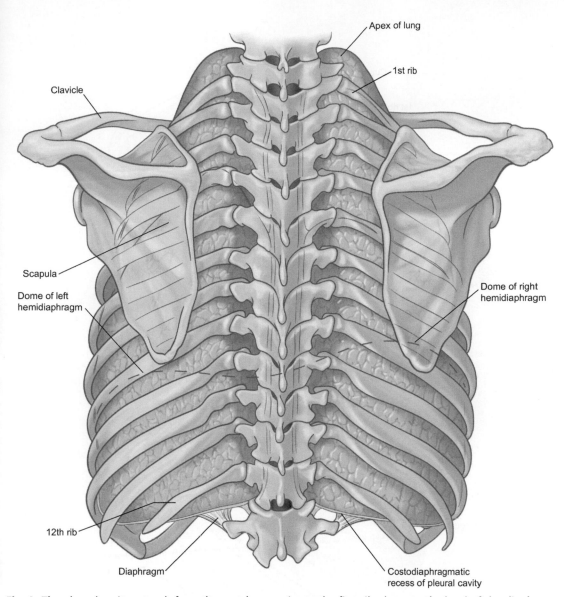

Fig. 4. The pleural cavity extends from the cupola, superior to the first rib, down to the level of the diaphragm.

pleural space into the lymphatic channels. These drain, depending on their location within the chest, to the diaphragmatic, internal mammary, retrosternal, paraesophageal, and even celiac lymph node stations.[15] Transdiaphragmatic channels also seem to be present, which may account for seeding of the pleural space by some abdominal malignancies.

NERVE SUPPLY

The parietal pleura has a rich supply of nervous innervation, including somatic, sympathetic, and parasympathetic fibers. These fibers are supplied via the intercostal nerves and were believed to be the only innervation of the pleura. However, recent evidence shows what seem to be nerve endings found within the visceral pleura in various animal species. Pintelon and colleagues[18] showed nerve fibers that are intimately associated with the elastic fibers of the lung, and are referred to as *visceral pleura receptors* (VPRs). VPRs are believed to mediate sensory transduction of painful or mechanical stimuli, and may be involved in the reflexive dyspnea that is seen in some pleural diseases.

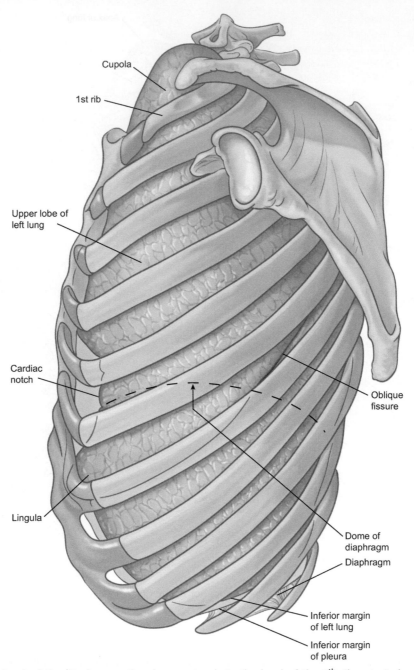

Fig. 5. At the level of the diaphragm, the pleura extends to the level of the 6th rib anteriorly and sometimes below the 12th rib posteriorly.

SUMMARY

The lung is encased in the thoracic cavity, a rigid structure that provides it with support and protection. The visceral and parietal pleura form the pleura cavity, which lines the lung parenchyma and inner aspect of the chest wall, respectively. The pleura allows the lung to move, with minimal friction, within the thoracic cavity. It also transmits the mechanical forces produced by the diaphragm and chest wall, allowing the lung to expand and contract. Fluid, cellular debris, and protein are cleared from the pleural space mainly through stomata, which are direct openings into the lymphatic channels through the mesothelial layer.

With a rich blood supply and lymphatic system just deep to the mesothelial layer, the pleura is a dynamic layer that protects the lung and pleural cavity from infection while transmitting the forces of respiration without damage to the underlying lung.

REFERENCES

1. D'Angelo E, Loring SH, Gioia ME, et al. Friction and lubrication of pleural tissues. Respir Physiol Neurobiol 2004;142:55.

2. Wang NS. Anatomy of the pleura. Clin Chest Med 1998;19:229.

3. Michailova KN. Ultrastructural observations on the human visceral pleura. Eur J Morphol 1997;35:125.

4. Wang NS. Anatomy and physiology of the pleural space. Clin Chest Med 1985;6:3.

5. Morrissey BM, Bisset RA. The right inferior lung margin: anatomy and clinical implication. Br J Radiol 1993;66:503.

6. Wang PM, Lai-Fook SJ. Regional pleural filtration and absorption measured by fluorescent tracers in rabbits. Lung 1999;177:289.

7. Li J. Ultrastructural study on the pleural stomata in human. Funct Dev Morphol 1993;3:277.

8. McLaughlin RF, Tyler WS, Canada RO. A study of the subgross pulmonary anatomy in various mammals. Am J Anat 1961;108:149–65.

9. McLaughlin RF. Bronchial artery distribution in various mammals and in humans. Am Rev Respir Dis 1983;128:S57.

10. Albertine KH, Wiener-Kronish JP, Roos PJ, et al. Structure, blood supply, and lymphatic vessels of the sheep's visceral pleura. Am J Anat 1982;165:277.

11. Gilbert E, Hakim TS. Relative contribution of bronchial flow to subpleural region in dog lung. J Appl Physiol 1992;73:855.

12. Wang PM, Lai-Fook SJ. Effect of ventilation frequency and tidal volume on pleural space thickness in rabbits. J Appl Physiol 1996;75:1836.

13. Zocchi L. Physiology and pathophysiology of pleural fluid turnover. Eur Respir J 2002;20:1545.

14. Miura T, Shimada T, Tanaka K, et al. Lymphatic drainage of carbon particles injected into the pleural cavity of the monkey, as studied by video-assisted thoracoscopy and electron microscopy. J Thorac Cardiovasc Surg 2000;120:437.

15. Okiemy G, Foucault C, Avisse C, et al. Lymphatic drainage of the diaphragmatic pleura to the peritracheobronchial lymph nodes. Surg Radiol Anat 2003;25:32.

16. Shinohara H. Distribution of lymphatic stomata on the pleural surface of the thoracic cavity and the surface topography of the pleural mesothelium in the golden hamster. Anat Rec 1997;249:16.

17. Riquet M, Badoual C, Le Pimpec Barthes F, et al. Visceral pleura invasion and pleural lavage tumor cytology by lung cancer: a prospective appraisal. Ann Thorac Surg 2003;75:353.

18. Pintelon I, Brouns I, De Proost I, et al. Sensory receptors in the visceral pleura: neurochemical coding and live staining in whole mounts. Am J Respir Cell Mol Biol 2007;36:541.

Anatomy of the Pleura: Reflection Lines and Recesses

François Bertin, MD[a], Jean Deslauriers, MD, FRCS(C)[b],*

KEYWORDS

- Anatomy • Pleural reflection lines • Pleural recesses

The pleura is made of 2 serosal membranes, one covering the lung (the visceral pleura) and one covering the inner chest wall (the parietal pleura). Their surfaces glide over each other, facilitating proper lung movements during the various phases of respiration. The transition between the parietal and visceral pleura is at the pulmonary hilum or root of the lung. At this level, the reflection covers the constituents of the hilum, except inferiorly, where the reflection extends down to the diaphragm and is called the triangular or inferior pulmonary ligament.

The parietal pleura is more complex anatomically than the visceral pleura, as it covers completely the inner surface of the thoracic wall through which it is attached via a fibrous layer known as the endothotracic fascia. The lines along which the parietal pleura changes direction as it passes from one wall of the pleural cavity to another are called the lines of pleural reflection. Because the lungs do not entirely fill the pleural spaces during expiration, the potential spaces thus created are called pleural recesses or sinuses. These recesses fill with lung during inspiration.

Before the advent of antituberculous drugs, the anatomy of pleural reflection lines and recesses was of great importance to all surgeons involved in the management of this disease, particularly those performing operations pertinent to collapse therapy such as extrapleural pneumonysis or apicolysis.[1–3] Currently, thorough knowledge of this anatomy is important for the correct interpretation of chest radiographs, as well as for the performance of procedures such as thoracentesis, tube drainage of the pleural space, or pericardiocentesis.

LINES OF PLEURAL REFLECTION AND TRIANGULAR LIGAMENTS

The lines of pleural reflection are formed by the parietal pleura as it changes direction (reflects) from one wall of the pleural cavity to another.

The sternal lines of reflection are where the costal parietal pleura becomes continuous with the mediastinal pleura. The external projection of those lines is fairly similar on both sides and extends from the level of the fourth costal cartilage on the left side and sixth costal cartilage on the right side to a point that lies approximately 3 to 4 cm above the anterior end of the first rib.

The costodiaphragmatic lines of reflection occur where the costal parietal pleura joins the diaphragmatic pleura inferiorly, and the vertebral lines of reflection run in the paravertebral planes from the first to the 12th thoracic vertebrae.

The parietal mediastinal pleura joins with the visceral pleura on the medial aspect of the lung at the level of the pulmonary hilum or root of the lung. Before joining the parietal pleural, the visceral pleura forms an almost circular sleeve that encloses the structures of the hilum (**Figs. 1** and **2**). Below the root, the reflection of the mediastinal pleura over the visceral pleura continues as a double layer of pleura in the front and back of the hilar plane. Together these 4 layers form a striplike fold that crosses in a slightly oblique direction,

[a] Service de Chirurgie Thoracique et Cardiovasculaire, CHU Dupuytren, Limoges, France
[b] Institut Universitaire de Cardiologie et de Pneumologie de Québec, Laval University, 2725 Chemin Sainte-Foy, Quebec City, Quebec G1V 4G5, Canada
* Corresponding author.
E-mail address: jean.deslauriers@chg.ulaval.ca

Thorac Surg Clin 21 (2011) 165–171
doi:10.1016/j.thorsurg.2010.12.002
1547-4127/11/$ – see front matter © 2011 Elsevier Inc. All rights reserved.

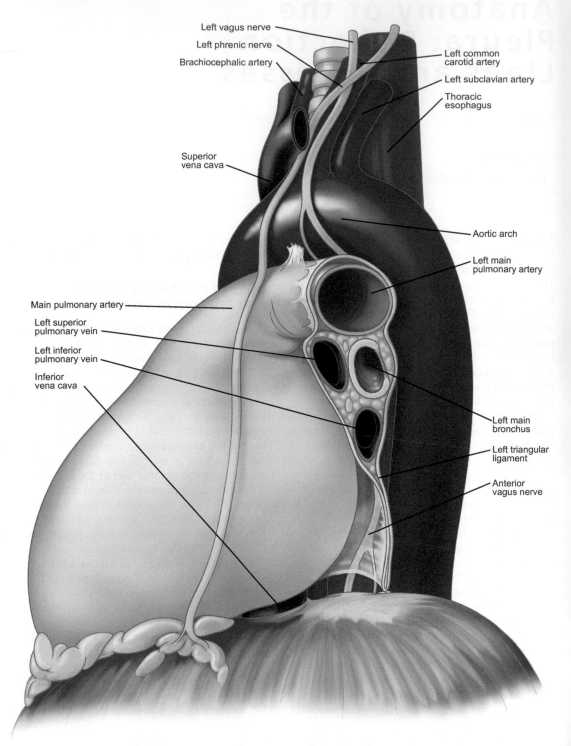

Left vagus nerve
Left phrenic nerve
Brachiocephalic artery
Left common carotid artery
Left subclavian artery
Thoracic esophagus
Superior vena cava
Aortic arch
Left main pulmonary artery
Main pulmonary artery
Left superior pulmonary vein
Left inferior pulmonary vein
Inferior vena cava
Left main bronchus
Left triangular ligament
Anterior vagus nerve

Fig. 1. Lateral view of the left hilum showing the anatomy of the left inferior pulmonary ligament (triangular ligament).

downwards and backwards. This fold of pleura, which stretches tightly from the medial aspect of the lung to the mediastinum, is called the triangular ligament of the lung or pulmonary ligament (ligamentum pulmonale) (see **Figs. 1** and **2**).

Each triangular ligament has an internal border, an external border, a lower border, and an apex. The internal border corresponds to the mediastinal pleura, which on the right side is inserted along the right lateral border of the esophagus (**Fig. 3**) and on

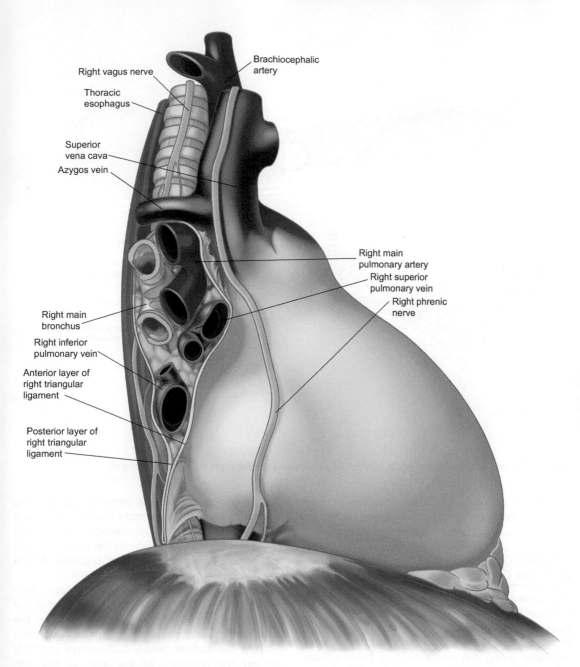

Fig. 2. Lateral view of the right hilum showing the anatomy of the right inferior pulmonary ligament (triangular ligament).

the left side on the posterior aspect of the pericardium and thoracic aorta. The external border corresponds to the mediastinal aspects of the lower lobes below the hilum. The lower border is located posteriorly, has a variable configuration, and can or not insert on the diaphragm. The apex of the pulmonary ligament reflects over the inferior pulmonary vein.

The space between the front and back layers of the triangular ligament contains loose connective tissue, small branches of bronchial and esophageal arteries, a few venules emptying into the superior diaphragmatic veins, and scattered lymphatic trunks and nodes draining the lower lobes of the lung and lower third of the thoracic esophagus.

PLEURAL RECESSES (RECESSUS PLEURALIS)

The junctions between the different segments of parietal pleura (costal, diaphragmatic, mediastinal) form several recesses that include on each side

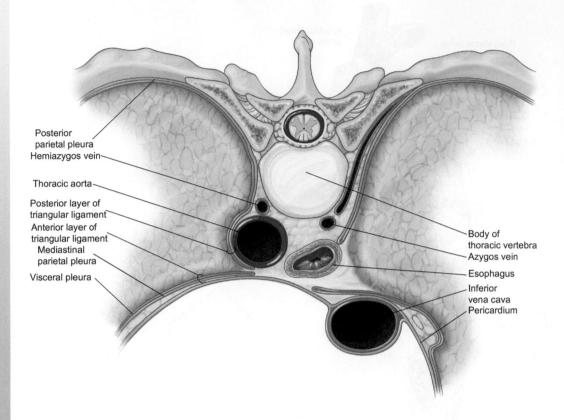

Posterior parietal pleura
Hemiazygos vein
Thoracic aorta
Posterior layer of triangular ligament
Anterior layer of triangular ligament
Mediastinal parietal pleura
Visceral pleura

Body of thoracic vertebra
Azygos vein
Esophagus
Inferior vena cava
Pericardium

Fig. 3. Diagram showing the pleural reflections at the level of the right triangular ligament.

a posterior and anterior costomediastinal recess, a mediastinodiaphragmatic recess, and an inferior or costodiaphragmatic recess.

Posterior Costomediastinal Recesses (Recesses Costomediastinalis)

The posterior costomediastinal recesses are at the junction between the mediastinal pleura and the posterior part of the costal pleura. They open in a forward and outward direction and they extend vertically along the costovertebral gutters from the first rib to the 11th intercostal space.

The anatomical relationships of these recesses are with the costovertebral junctions, the origin of posterior intercostal arteries and intercostal nerves, the sympathetic chains, and the azygos venous system (azygos vein on the right side and hemiazygos vein on the left side).

Anterior Costomediastinal Recesses

The anterior costomediastinal recesses are the junction between the mediastinal pleura and the anterior part of the costal pleura. They are narrower and deeper than their posterior counterpart

and they extend from the sternoclavicular joints superiorly to the seventh costal cartilages inferiorly (**Fig. 4**). The anterior costomediastinal recesses are different from one side to the other, the left recess being potentially larger because of the cardiac notch in the left lung.

On the right side, the anterior costomediastinal recess has a rounded externally concave shape. From the sternoclavicular joint to the level of the second costal cartilage, it is directed toward the midline before descending vertically behind the sternum. At the level of the fifth intercostal space, it turns downward and to the right (away from the midline) until it reaches the seventh costal cartilage where it is in continuity with the costodiaphragmatic recess.

On the left side, the contours of the anterior costomediastinal recess are symmetrical to those on the right side from the sternoclavicular joint to the second costal cartilage. From that point, it courses vertically to the left of the midline down to the level of the fourth costal cartilage where it diverges obliquely and outward so that it is about 3 cm from the midline upon reaching the costodiaphragmatic recess at the level of the seventh costal cartilage.

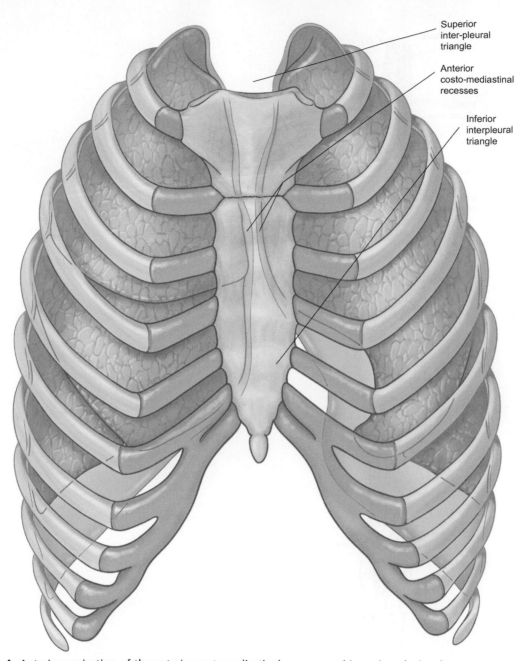

Superior
inter-pleural
triangle

Anterior
costo-mediastinal
recesses

Inferior
interpleural
triangle

Fig. 4. Anterior projection of the anterior costomediastinal recesses and interpleural triangles.

The contours of the right and left anterior costo-mediastinal recesses form 2 interpleural triangles, a superior one with an apex pointing downward, and an inferior one with an apex pointing upward (see **Fig. 4**). This configuration explains why the anterior mediastinum can be surgically accessed via a median sternotomy without entering the pleural spaces.

Ventrally, the anatomical relationships of the anterior costomediastinal recesses are with the sternocostal plate, the anterior ends of the costal

cartilages and intercostal spaces, and the internal mammary blood vessels. Dorsally, the anterior costomediastinal recesses are in relation with the thymus superiorly and the pericardium inferiorly.

Mediastinodiaphragmatic Recesses (Recessus Mediastino Diaphragmaticus)

The mediastinodiaphragmatic recesses are at the junction between the mediastinal pleura and the diaphragmatic pleura. They are widely opened in

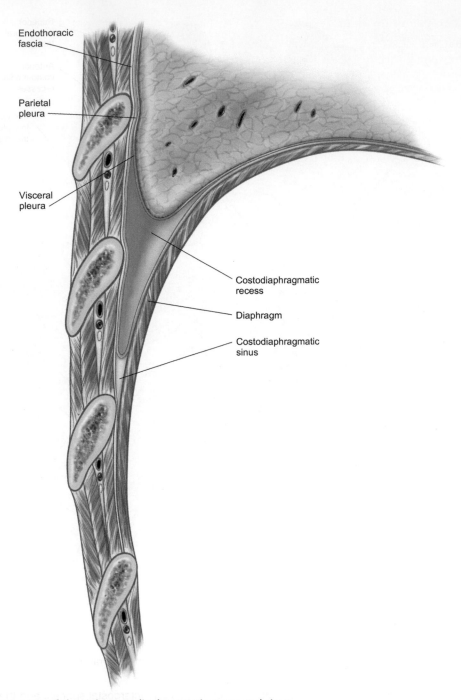

Endothoracic fascia

Parietal pleura

Visceral pleura

Costodiaphragmatic recess

Diaphragm

Costodiaphragmatic sinus

Fig. 5. Projection of the right costodiaphragmatic recess and sinus.

an upward and outward direction and they extend from the posterior aspect of the sternum to the posterior end of the 11th intercostal space.

The anatomical relationships of the mediastinodiaphragmatic recesses are different on the right and left sides. On the right, the pericardium and right phrenic nerve separate the recess from the right atrium and inferior vena cava and the recess is also in relation with the right border of the esophagus and right vagus nerve. On the left side, the pericardium and left phrenic nerve separate the recess from the left ventricle and more dorsally from the esophagus and left vagus nerve. The left mediastinodiaphragmatic recess is also in relation with the descending thoracic aorta.

Costodiaphragmatic Recesses (Recessus Costodiaphragmaticus)

The costodiaphragmatic recesses (**Fig. 5**) are at the junction between the costal and diaphragmatic pleura. They extend from the the seventh costal cartilage anteriorly to the neck of the 12th rib posteriorly. Their course is obliquely downward and to the back. They follow but never quite reach the bottom of the costodiaphragmatic sinuses from which they are separated by a layer of subpleural tissue of variable density.

Through the diaphragm, the costodiaphragmatic recesses are in relation with several intra-abdominal structures such as the convexity of the liver on the right side and the spleen and greater tuberosity of the stomach on the left. On both sides, the recesses are in relation with the perirenal spaces, the posterior aspects of the kidneys, and the adrenal glands that project in front of the 11th rib.

Posteriorly, the anatomical relationships of the costodiaphragmatic recesses with the 12th rib are variable and depend on the length of the rib. If the rib is short, it will be almost totally covered by the recess but if, on the other hand, the rib is long, it will be crossed by the recess at a distance of approximately 7 cm from the midline.

SUMMARY

Knowledge of the anatomy of the lines of pleural reflection, triangular ligaments, and pleural recesses is important to thoracic surgeons because their anatomic areas are used daily for radiographic interpretation as well as for the performance of procedures such as chest tube insertion, thoracentesis, and pericardiocentesis. Their knowledge is also important for thoracic surgeons doing surgical procedures, such as parietal pleurectomies, extrapleural mobilization and resection of the lungs, and pleuroneumonectomies for destroyed lungs or malignant pleural neoplasms.

ACKNOWLEDGMENTS

The authors thank Dr Jerôme Cau for his technical assistance and Andrew Corsini for proofreading and translating the manuscript.

REFERENCES

1. Dungan DJ, Samson PC. Surgical significance of the endothoracic fascia. The anatomic basis for empyemectomy and other extrapleural techniques. Am J Surg 1975;130:151–8.
2. Eloesser L, Brown PK. Surgical intervention in pulmonary tuberculosis. Am Rev Tuberc 1924;8:519.
3. Alexander J. The collapse therapy of tuberculosis. Springfield (IL): Thomas; 1937.

FURTHER READINGS

Bouchet A, Cuilleret J. Anatomie topographique, descriptive et fonctionnelle: Le cou, le thorax. 2nd édition. Paris: Simep; 1991.

Cordier GJ, Cabrol C. Les pédicules segmentaires du poumon: Le poumon droit. Paris: Expansion Scientifique Française; 1952.

Cordier GJ, Cabrol C. Les pédicules segmentaires du poumon: Le poumon gauche. Paris: Expansion Scientifique Française; 1952.

Gray H. Gray's anatomy. The anatomical basis of clinical practice. 39th edition. Philadelphia: Elsevier; 2005.

Moore KL, Dalley AF. Clinically oriented anatomy. 5th edition. Philadelphia: Lippincott, Williams, Wilkins; 2005. p. 116–7.

Microscopic Anatomy of the Pleura

Carla M. Sevin, MD*, Richard W. Light, MD

KEYWORDS

- Pleura • Blood supply • Lymphatics • Pleural fluid

The pleura consists of two components: the parietal pleura, which lines the inside of the thoracic cavities, and the visceral pleura, which covers the lung parenchyma. These develop from the same serous membrane, merge at the hilum, and differ only in the structures they cover.

Microscopically, the pleura is made up of five different layers. The layer adjacent to the pleural space is made up of a single layer of mesothelial cells. Beneath these cells lies a thin layer of connective tissue, a superficial elastic layer, a loose, irregular connective tissue layer containing adipose tissue, vessels, nerves, and lymphatics, and a deep fibroelastic layer adhering to the underlying structure (lung, mediastinum, diaphragm, or chest wall). In the parietal pleura, this fifth layer is also known as the endothoracic fascia.[1]

The thickness of each layer varies among species and even within one organism. The visceral pleura is generally thin near the apex, with flattened mesothelial cells that have sparse microvilli. Towards the base of the lung the pleura becomes thicker and the mesothelial cells more cuboidal in shape; the number of microvilli increases, facilitating the active movement and stretching of this portion of the lung.[2]

BLOOD SUPPLY

The blood supply to the visceral pleura depends on its thickness. In animals with thick visceral pleura, the blood supply is predominantly from the systemic circulation. If the visceral pleura is thin, the blood supply is drawn mainly from the pulmonary circulation (ie, the bronchial arteries).[3] Humans have a relatively thick visceral pleura, and it is generally agreed that most, if not all, of the visceral pleura in humans is supplied by the bronchial artery.[4] Venous drainage is via the pulmonary veins.

The parietal pleura is supplied by systemic capillaries. The pericardiacophrenic artery is the principal blood supply for the mediastinal pleura. On the chest wall, small intercostal artery branches supply the costal pleura. Over the diaphragm, the pleura is supplied by the superior phrenic and musculophrenic arteries. Venous drainage is primarily via the intercostal veins. Blood from the diaphragmatic pleura drains caudally via the inferior phrenic veins or cranially via the superior phrenic veins.[4]

LYMPHATICS

The visceral pleura has an extensive lymphatic system, but it does not connect to the pleural space.[3] The lymphatic vessels of the parietal and diaphragmatic pleura, however, do connect to the pleural space via stomata, tiny holes 8 μm to 10 μm in diameter formed by discontinuities in the mesothelial layer, where it abuts the underlying lymphatic endothelium (**Fig. 1**).[5,6] These lymphatics are the major route by which liquid exits the pleural space. From the stomata, liquid drains to the lacunae, a lacey collection of submesothelial lymphatics, and from there to infracostal lymphatics, parasternal and periaortic nodes, thoracic duct, and eventually into the systemic venous system.

In a study of lymph nodes draining the pleural space in pigs and rats, Parungo and colleagues found that injections of a lymph tracer into the pleural space drained solely to the highest superior mediastinal lymph node group (lymph node

Department of Medicine, Division of Allergy, Pulmonary and Critical Care Medicine, Vanderbilt University Medical Center, 1161 21st Avenue South, T-1218 Medical Center North, Nashville, TN 37232-2640, USA
* Corresponding author.
E-mail address: carla.sevin@vanderbilt.edu

Thorac Surg Clin 21 (2011) 173–175
doi:10.1016/j.thorsurg.2010.12.003

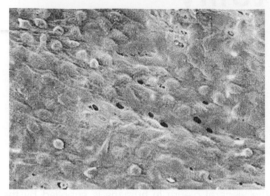

Fig. 1. Scanning electron micrograph of a group of stomata in the anterior lower chest of a rat. The surrounding depression is probably the boundary of a lacuna, a cystic dilated lymphatic space beneath the pleura (magnified 1500×). (*Reproduced from* Wang NS. Anatomy of the Pleura. Clin Chest Med 1998;19:236; with permission.)

station 1), suggesting that these are the sentinel lymph nodes of the pleural space.[7]

PLEURAL FLUID

Normally the amount of pleural fluid is small; less than 1 mL can be collected from the pleural cavity of a person unaffected by disease. It arises from systemic pleural vessels, moves slowly across leaky pleural membranes into the pleural space, and exits this space via the pleural lymphatic system described previously.[8]

Pleural fluid forms a thin layer between the visceral and parietal pleurae and appears to be relatively evenly distributed in this space. This fluid prevents contact between the visceral and parietal surfaces, and keeps frictional forces between the lungs and chest wall low.[9]

In the absence of disease, the mean white cell count in human pleural fluid is 1716 cells/mm[3], and the mean red cell count is about 700 cells/mm[3]. A normal differential is about 75% macrophages, 25% lymphocytes, and less than 2% each mesothelial cells, neutrophils, and eosinophils.[10]

MESOTHELIAL CELLS

In people, the mesothelial cell ranges from 16.4 plus or minus 6.8 μm to 41.9 plus or minus 9.5 μm in diameter, and from less than 1 μm to greater than 4 μm in thickness.[2,3] Its shape and size tends to reflect the structure it covers; the mesothelial cell may appear flattened or cuboidal. Mesothelial cells are frequently dislodged from their surfaces and float freely in the pleural fluid, where their shape becomes round or oval.

A tight junction joins the cells at the apical portion of the mesothelial layer. However, at other junctions the cells may overlap without being attached to each other. The overlap disappears with deep inspiration. The junctional complexes between mesothelial cell membranes are loose, similar to the endothelium in the venous system. However, these interactions are more complex among visceral mesothelial cells compared with parietal ones, suggesting that the visceral layer is less leaky or subject to more stretch than the parietal side.[2]

The mesothelial cell surface is unevenly covered with bushy microvilli (**Figs. 2** and **3**). These microvilli are approximately 0.1 μm in diameter and 0.5 μm to 3 μm in length, and are most numerous over the inferior visceral pleura and on the anterior and inferior mediastinal surfaces of the parietal pleura.[2] Their density may range from a few to more than 600 per 100 μm[2]. More microvilli are found on the visceral pleura than on corresponding regions of the parietal pleura.

The exact function of mesothelial microvilli has not been defined. However, it is thought that their most important function is to enmesh glycoproteins rich in hyaluronic acid, in order to lessen the friction between the lung and thorax.[2] Hyaluronic acid is secreted by mesothelial cells and by mesenchymal cells in the subpleural space.

Numerous pinocytic vesicles are found at the pleural and basal cell membranes of pleural mesothelial cells. The ovoid nucleus often has a prominent nucleolus. The thickness of the cytoplasm varies, but always exhibits many well developed organelles, suggesting it is a metabolically active cell.[2] When free floating in the pleural fluid, the mesothelial cell can be transformed into a macrophage capable of phagocytosis and

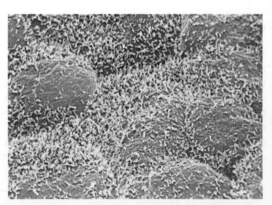

Fig. 2. Scanning electron micrograph showing parietal pleural mesothelial cells with a dense population of microvilli (rabbit, magnified 1300×). (*Reproduced from* Wang NS. Anatomy of the Pleura. Clin Chest Med 1998;19:231; with permission.)

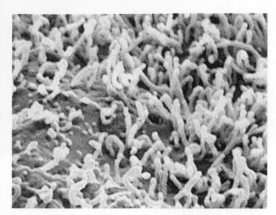

Fig. 3. A close-up view of surface microvilli of a meso-thelial cell. Scanning electron micrograph, parietal pleura (rabbit, magnified 13,000×). (*Reproduced from* Wang NS. Anatomy of the Pleura. Clin Chest Med 1998;19:232; with permission.)

erythrophagocytosis.[11] There is also evidence that mesothelial cells can convert to myofibroblasts.[12]

The mesothelial layer is very fragile. When disrupted, the defect is repaired via mitosis and migration of the mesothelial cells.[13] Irritated mesothelial cells retract but maintain their continuity with adjacent cells via projections known as cellular bridges.

KAMPMEIER FOCI

Irregular elevated foci consisting of microscopic aggregates of lymphocytes, histiocytes, plasma cells, and other mononuclear cells around central lymphatic or vascular vessels have been found on the pleura and mesentery of many species of mammals. First described in 1863 by von Recklinghausen in rabbits and later by Kampmeier as small pleural milky spots on the mediastina of rats and humans, these foci are thought to function like enlarged lymphoid tissues.[2] Intrapleural instillation of immunomodulatory agents causes an increase in size and cellularity of these milky spots, whereas steroids induce a slight atrophy.[14] These experimental results suggest that Kampmeier spots play a role in inflammatory and immune responses in the pleural space.

REFERENCES

1. Light RW. Anatomy of the Pleura. In: Pleural diseases. 5th edition. Philadelphia: Lippincott Williams & Wilkins; 2007. p. 1–6.
2. Wang NS. Anatomy of the pleura. Clin Chest Med 1998;19:229–40.
3. Albertine KH, Wiener-Kronish JP, Roos PJ, et al. Structure, blood supply, and lymphatic vessels of the sheep's visceral pleura. Am J Anat 1982;165:277–94.
4. Peng MJ, Wang NS. Embryology and gross structure. In: Light R, Lee YC, editors. Textbook of pleural diseases. 3rd edition. London: Arnold Publishing; 2003. p. 3–16.
5. Wang NS. The preformed stomas connecting the pleural cavity and the lymphatics in the parietal pleura. Am Rev Respir Dis 1975;111:12–20.
6. Li J. Ultrastructural study on the pleural stomata in human. Funct Dev Morphol 1993;3:277–80.
7. Parungo CP, Colson YL, Kim SW, et al. Sentinel lymph node mapping of the pleural space. Chest 2005;127(5):1799–804.
8. Broaddus VC, Light RW. Pleural effusion. In: Mason RJ, Broaddus VC, Murray JF, et al, editors. Murray and Nadel's textbook of respiratory medicine. 4th edition. Philadelphia: Elsevier; 2005. p. 1913–60.
9. Albertine KH, Wiener-Kronish JP, Bastacky J, et al. No evidence for mesothelial cell contact across the costal pleural space of sheep. J Appl Physiol 1991;70:123–43.
10. Noppen M, De Waele M, Li R, et al. Volume and cellular content of normal pleural fluid in humans examined by pleural lavage. Am J Respir Crit Care Med 2000;162(3):1023–6.
11. Bakalos D, Constantakis N, Isicricas T. Distinction of mononuclear macrophages from mesothelial cells in pleural and peritoneal effusions. Acta Cytol 1974; 18(1):20–2.
12. Yang AH, Chen JY, Lin JK. Myofibroblastic conversion of mesothelial cells. Kidney Int 2003;63(4):1530–9.
13. Peng MJ, Wang NS, Vargas FS, et al. Subclinical surface alterations of human pleura. Chest 1994; 106:351–3.
14. Pereira AD, Aguas AP, Oliveira MJ, et al. Experimental modulation of the reactivity of pleural milky spots (Kampmeier's foci) by Freund's adjuvants, betamethasone and mycobacterial infection. J Anat 1994;185:471–9.

Correlative Anatomy of the Pleura and Pleural Spaces

Chen Liang, MD[a], Li Shuang, MD[a], Liu Wei, MD[b],
Jean-Philippe Bolduc, MD[c], Jean Deslauriers, MD, FRCS(C)[d],*

KEYWORDS

- Pleura • Pleural space • Anatomy

Pathologic processes involving the pleura and the pleural spaces are often complex and are sometimes difficult to diagnose and manage.[1] Intimate knowledge of the normal anatomy of the pleura and, most importantly, of the correlation between anatomy and imaging is thus important for anyone, especially thoracic surgeons, involved in the diagnosis and management of these diseases.

Although the parietal and visceral layers of the pleura are seldom seen on standard chest films because their shadows blend with other densities, such as those of the chest wall, mediastinum, and diaphragm, conventional radiographs remain the basic imaging modality for the initial assessment of patients suspected of having a pleural disorder. It is simple, accessible, safe, cheap, and fast in addition to allowing for bedside examination. Depending on the clinical context, further evaluation can be done through several other imaging modalities, such as conventional or high-resolution CT.[2] These techniques have a greater sensitivity to characterize the pleural anatomy and the excellent spatial resolution now possible from multi-detector CT scanning has further improved the depiction of all anatomic regions of the pleural space.[3]

The role of MRI is currently more limited not only because the normal pleural space cannot be visualized with MRI techniques[4] but also because the diagnostic capabilities of MRI are largely similar to those of CT.

NORMAL ANATOMY OF THE PLEURA AND PLEURAL SPACES

The pleura is made of 2 serous membranes: one covering the inner chest wall, which is called the parietal pleura, and one covering the lung surface, which is called the visceral pleura. The transition between the 2 membranes is at the level of the hilum where the pleural reflection covers the constituents of the lung root, except inferiorly where it extends down to the diaphragm to form the inferior pulmonary ligament.

The visceral pleura covers the outer surface of the lung and extends into the fissures to cover each individual lobe. It is thin, transparent, and tightly adherent to the underlying lung.

The parietal pleura is usually divided into costal, mediastinal, and diaphragmatic segments. At the level of the chest wall, the parietal pleura is attached to the bony thorax through a fibrous layer known as the endothoracic fascia. The presence of this fascia provides a plane of dissection that makes it easy for surgeons to perform a parietal pleurectomy. The transition between each

[a] Department of Radiology, First Teaching Hospital of Jilin University, Changchun, Jilin Province, People's Republic of China
[b] Department of Thoracic Surgery, First Teaching Hospital of Jilin University, Changhun, Jilin Province, People's Republic of China
[c] Department of Radiology, Institut Universitaire de Cardiologie et de Pneumologie de Québec, Canada
[d] Institut Universitaire de Cardiologie et de Pneumologie de Québec, Laval University, 2725 Chemin Sainte-Foy, Quebec City, Quebec G1V 4G5, Canada
* Corresponding author.
E-mail address: jean.deslauriers@chg.ulaval.ca

Thorac Surg Clin 21 (2011) 177–182
doi:10.1016/j.thorsurg.2010.12.006
1547-4127/11/$ – see front matter © 2011 Elsevier Inc. All rights reserved.

segment of parietal pleura is at the level of the pleural sinuses.

IMAGING OF THE VISCERAL PLEURA AND LUNG FISSURES

On standard posteroanterior (PA) and lateral chest films, the visceral pleura appears as a hairline of soft-tissue density not clearly defined because it is obscured by the shadows of the ribs and soft tissues of the chest wall.

At the interfaces between the various lobes, the visceral pleura extends down into the interlobar fissures. These fissures are important radiological landmarks and their recognition is useful to accurately localize and analyze pulmonary disease processes.[5] On standard radiographs fissures are seen as thin hyperattenuating lines. On the right side, the major oblique fissure separates the lower lobe from the upper and middle lobe and the minor fissure, which is less well developed, runs horizontally to separate the upper lobe from the middle lobe; whereas, on the left side, the major oblique fissure separates the lower lobe from the upper lobe. Both oblique fissures run from the level of T_3 posteriorly to the level of the sixth costochondral junction anteriorly. They have a gently curved surface where the upper part of the fissure is concave anteriorly and faces laterally; whereas, the lower part is convex anteriorly and faces medially.[6] On PA frontal standard radiographs, oblique fissures are normally invisible because they are not tangent to the x-ray beam. Portions of these fissures can, however, be delineated on lateral roentgenograms (**Fig. 1**) when they become tangent to the x-ray beam. The left oblique fissure is generally more posterior than the right oblique fissure, which can also be identified when its junction with the minor horizontal fissure is demonstrable (**Fig. 2**). The oblique fissures are seldom seen in their totality either because they are anatomically incomplete or are obscured by the superimposition of structures.

The minor horizontal fissure, which separates the right upper lobe from the middle lobe, begins at the oblique fissure in the midaxillary line at the level of the fifth or sixth rib and runs transversely to the fourth costal cartilage. On a lateral radiograph, it can be seen in more than half of normal individuals (see **Fig. 2**) and it is not truly horizontal but gently curved with its convexity upward.

On conventional CT, major fissures are almost always identified[7] and they show as avascular zones of decreased attenuation along the interfaces between lobes (**Fig. 3**), as lines, or less often as dense bands. On high-resolution CT, major fissures most often appear as sharp lines (**Fig. 4**).[6] On the right side, the minor fissure can be identified as a triangular hypovascular area lateral to the bronchus intermedius,[5,8] with its apex at the hilar region.

Accessory fissures between pulmonary segments are not uncommon and can often be recognized radiographically. Anatomically, these are clefts of varying depth lined by 2 layers of visceral pleura.[9] The best known of these accessory fissures is the azygos fissure (seen in 1% of normal individuals), which separates a variable portion of the medial right upper lobe from the rest of the lobe, with the azygos vein coursing in the fissure's inferior extent (**Fig. 5**). Other less common accessory fissures include an inferior

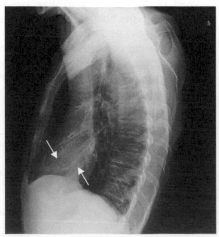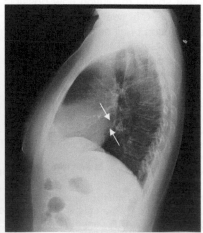

Fig. 1. Normal radiological anatomy of major fissures. Lateral chest radiographs showing the right (*1.1*) and left major fissures (*1.2*); note that the fissures are seen as double lines and that the left oblique fissure is located behind the right one (*arrow, 1.2*).

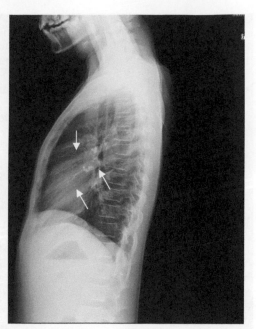

Fig. 2. Lateral chest radiograph showing the horizontal fissure (*1 arrow*) and the right oblique fissure (*2 arrows*).

accessory fissure that separates the medial basal segment from the rest of the lower lobe (more common on the right side) and a left minor fissure that separates the lingula from the rest of the upper lobe. The recognition of these accessory fissures is helpful for segmental localization of pulmonary lesions, assessment of pulmonary disease processes, and assistance in differentiating

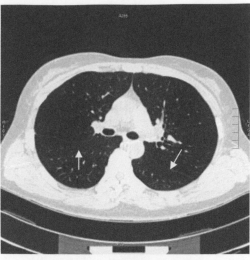

Fig. 4. High-resolution CT showing major fissures as dense lines (*arrows*).

accessory fissures from normal anatomical or pathological structures.[9,10]

The inferior pulmonary ligaments, which are a reflection of the mediastinal pleura around the pulmonary hilum, course inferoposterior from the inferior pulmonary veins.[3] When visible on CT, these ligaments are seen as short, thin lines or septa that extend laterally into the lung from the posterior mediastinal pleural margins. On the left, they are adjacent to or slightly anterior to the esophagus[3] (**Fig. 6**); whereas, on the right side

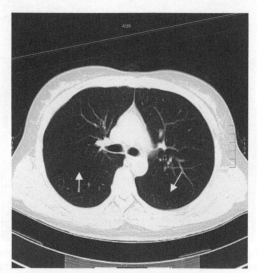

Fig. 3. CT scan depicting major fissures as avascular zones of decreased attenuation (*arrows*).

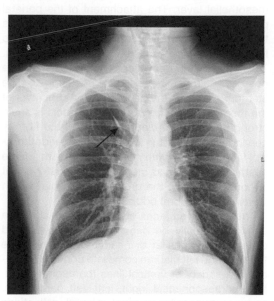

Fig. 5. Posteroanterior chest radiograph showing an azygos fissure (*arrow*) separating the medial aspect of the right upper lobe from the rest of the lobe.

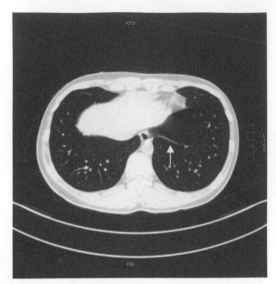

Fig. 6. CT scan showing the inferior pulmonary ligament as a thin line extending laterally from the lung (*arrow*).

they relate to the mediastinal aspect of the azygos vein.

IMAGING OF THE PARIETAL PLEURA

The parietal pleura has a thickness of approximately 100 to 200 μm (0.1 mm)[10] and it almost completely covers the inner surface of the thoracic wall and medial aspect of the mediastinum. It consists of 3 layers of tissue: a subpleural connective tissue layer, an elastic layer, and a parietal mesothelial layer. The attachment of the parietal pleura to the chest wall and mediastinum is through a fibrous layer, called the endothoracic fascia, with a thickness that varies with its location. The fascia is strongest over the inner surface of the ribs and almost nonexistent posterior to the sternum and over the pericardium. At the level of the thoracic inlet, the endothoracic fascia is again strong and forms a diaphragm called the fibrous cervicothoracic septum. Anteriorly, the endothoracic fascia blends with the perichondrium of the costal cartilages and sternum, and posteriorly it is continuous with the prevertebral fascia, which covers the vertebral bodies.[11]

The anterior surfaces of the mediastinal pleura can occasionally be demonstrated on standard chest radiographs at or near the midline where the right and left pleurae come into contact. Posteriorly, a variety of vertical lines (paraspinal [right, left], paraesophageal [right, left], left para-aortic, azygoesophageal) represent pleural reflections delineated by the presence of air in the adjacent lungs (**Fig. 7**).

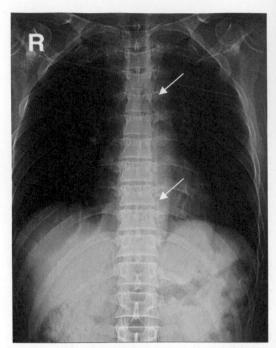

Fig. 7. PA chest radiograph showing a normal left paravertebral line (*arrows*).

On high-resolution CT, 1- to 2-mm thick lines of soft-tissue attenuation are visible over the anterolateral and posterolateral intercostal spaces and they represent the combined thickness of the visceral pleura, parietal pleura, endothoracic fascia, and innermost intercostals muscle (**Fig. 8**). These lines are easier to identify when

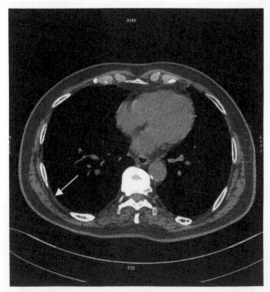

Fig. 8. High-resolution CT showing a 1- to 2-mm line representing the combined thickness of the visceral pleura, parietal pleura, endothoracic fascia, and innermost intercostal muscle (*arrow*).

they are outlined by air (**Fig. 9**) or fluid in the pleural space or when the parietal pleura is abnormally thickened (**Fig. 10**).

IMAGING OF THE LINES OF PLEURAL REFLECTION

Anatomical areas where the parietal pleura makes an abrupt change in its direction from one part of the pleural cavity to another are called lines of pleural reflection. Depending on their location, these lines are named sternal reflection line, costal reflection line, or vertebral reflection line.

Sternal reflection lines represent the junction between the costal pleura anteriorly and the mediastinal pleura. They extend from the sternoclavicular junctions cephalad in an almost vertical inferomedial direction to the sternal angle where both come in close contact. From that point, the right sternal reflection line extends downward and medially to the level of the xyphoid where it curves laterally. On the left side, it extends downward and medially to the level of the fourth costal cartilage. It then curves along the left sternal border and goes downward and obliquely to the level of the sixth costal cartilage. This particular anatomical arrangement creates an area where the pericardium is directly in contact with the anterior chest wall and where safe pericardiocentesis can be carried out.

The costal reflection lines correspond to areas where the costal pleura changes into diaphragmatic

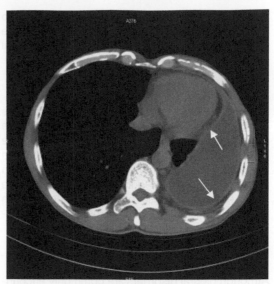

Fig. 10. CT scan of a patient with a pleural effusion showing abnormal thickening of both the visceral and parietal pleurae (*arrows*).

pleura. These lines are located at the level of the eighth rib at the midclavicular line, the 10th rib at the midaxillary line, and at the posterior portion of the 12th rib at the scapular line.

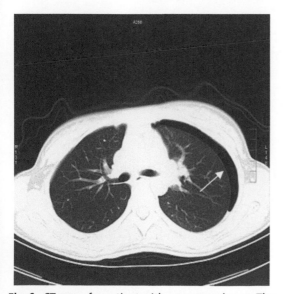

Fig. 9. CT scan of a patient with a pneumothorax. The visceral pleura is seen as a thin line over the lung (*arrow*); whereas, the parietal pleura is not well defined. Note that the visceral pleura margin follows the smooth and curved contour of the lung.

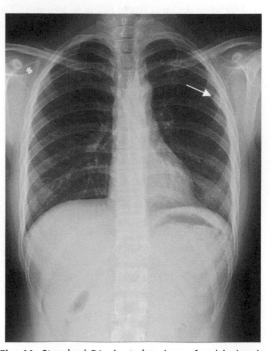

Fig. 11. Standard PA chest showing a focal lesion in the extrapleural space; note the well-defined margins of the lesion with an obtuse angle at the chest wall interface (*arrow*).

The vertebral reflection lines correspond to areas where the posterior costal pleura joins the mediastinal pleura parallel to the dorsal vertebral bodies.

IMAGING OF THE EXTRAPLEURAL SPACE

The extrapleural space is a virtual space that lies between the parietal pleura and the rib cage. The structures contained within that space include connective tissues, nerves, blood vessels, and muscles. With intact pleura overlying it, an abnormal lesion located in the extrapleural space will present an obtuse or tapering angle at the chest wall interface (**Fig. 11**) producing a characteristic shadow on standard radiographs.

SUMMARY

Although pleural disorders are commonly encountered in the daily practices of thoracic surgeons, their assessment can be difficult. Being able to correlate normal and abnormal anatomy with imaging characteristics provides additional information that can be useful not only to accurately locate pleuropulmonary lesions but also to characterize abnormalities, such as pleural thickening or malignant processes.

REFERENCES

1. Hierholzer J, Luo L, Bittner RC, et al. MRI and CT in the differential diagnosis of pleural disease. Chest 2000;118:604–9.
2. Müller NL. Imaging of the pleura. Radiology 1993; 186:297–309.
3. Gierada DS. Pleura imaging. In: Patterson GA, Cooper JD, Deslauriers J, et al, editors. Pearson's thoracic and esophageal surgery. 3rd edition. Philadelphia: Elsevier Inc; 2007. p. 1008–32.
4. McLoud TC, Flower CD. Imaging the pleura: sonography, CT, and MR Imaging. AJR Am J Roentgenol 1991;156:1145–53.
5. Proto AV, Ball JB. Computed tomography of the major and minor fissures. AJR 1983;140:439–48.
6. Hayashi K, Aziz A, Ashizawa K, et al. Radiographic and CT appearances of the major fissures. Radiographics 2001;21:861–74.
7. Sofranik RM, Gross BH, Spizarny DL. Radiology of the pleural fissures. Clin Imaging 1992;16:221–9.
8. Berkmen YM, Auh YH, Davis SD, et al. Anatomy of the minor fissure: evaluation with thin-section CT. Radiology 1989;170:647–51.
9. Yildiz A, Gölpinar F, Çalikõglu M, et al. HRCT evaluation of the accessory fissures of the lung. Eur J Radiol 2004;49:245–9.
10. Ariyürek OM, Gülsün M, Demirkasik FB. Accessory fissures of the lung: evaluation by high-resolution computed tomography. Eur Radiol 2001;11:2449–53.
11. Im JG, Webb WR, Rosen A, et al. Costal pleura: appearances at high-resolution CT. Radiology 1989;171:125–31.

FURTHER READING

Filsen B. Chest roentgenology. Philadelphia: WB Saunders Company; 1973.

Mediastinal Divisions and Compartments

Wei Liu, MD[a], Jean Deslauriers, MD, FRCS(C)[b],*

KEYWORDS
- Anatomy of the mediastinum • Mediastinal divisions
- Mediastinal compartments

The mediastinum (from the Greek *medium istemi*) is a complex anatomic region that extends from the thoracic inlet superiorly to the diaphragm inferiorly and from the posterior walls of the sternum and costal cartilages anteriorly to the thoracic vertebral bodies posteriorly. It is bordered laterally on each side by the mediastinal pleura. It is the central part of the thorax and major structures located or running through it include the trachea and main bronchi, the heart and great vessels, the esophagus, the thymus, and important segments of the lymphatic system.

Given the complexity of these structures, anatomists, clinicians, and radiologists have proposed dividing it into various compartments because such division is of practical value whenever one is elaborating a differential diagnosis or selecting the best surgical approach for a mediastinal mass or abnormality. Although numerous arbitrary divisions have been advocated over the years, most surgical textbooks adhere to the classic Gray's classification[1] of 4 compartments even if the most useful for thoracic surgeons are probably the 3-compartment model and Shields' 3-zone classification.[2]

COMPARTMENTS OF THE MEDIASTINUM
Four-Compartment Scheme

The most classic and probably oldest description of mediastinal compartments is the one suggested in Gray's anatomy textbook[1] in which the mediastinum is divided into 4 subdivisions: superior, anterior, middle, and posterior (**Fig. 1**; **Table 1**).

In that scheme, the superior mediastinum originates at the thoracic inlet[3] and extends inferiorly to a horizontal plane established by a virtual line drawn between the sterno-manubrial junction (angle de Louis) in the front and the lower part of the fourth thoracic vertebra (T4) in the back. This compartment contains all of the structures traversing the thoracic inlet, including the aorta and its major branches, the intrathoracic trachea, the upper third of the thoracic esophagus, the upper half of the superior vena cava, and the upper poles of the thymus.

The anterior mediastinum (antero-inferior), which is the smallest of this 4-compartment scheme, is located between the body of the sternum in the front and the anterior pericardium posteriorly. It contains loose connective tissues, mediastinal fat, and the body of the thymus, which is prominent during childhood but becomes atrophic in the adult.

The middle mediastinum is bounded anteriorly and posteriorly by the pericardium (see **Fig. 1**) and it contains the pericardium itself, the intrapericardial cardiovascular structures, the carina and main bronchi, and important lymph nodes and collecting lymph trunks located at and around the carina.

The posterior mediastinum extends from the dorsal surfaces of the pericardium, tracheal bifurcation, and main pulmonary blood vessels to the ventral surface of the lower 8 thoracic vertebrae. It

[a] Thoracic Surgical Service, First Teaching Hospital of Jilin University, Changchun, People's Republic of China
[b] Institut Universitaire de Cardiologie et de Pneumologie de Québec, Laval University, 2725 Chemin Sainte-Foy, Quebec City, Quebec G1V 4G5, Canada
* Corresponding author.
E-mail address: jean.deslauriers@chg.ulaval.ca

Thorac Surg Clin 21 (2011) 183–190
doi:10.1016/j.thorsurg.2010.12.005
1547-4127/11/$ – see front matter © 2011 Elsevier Inc. All rights reserved.

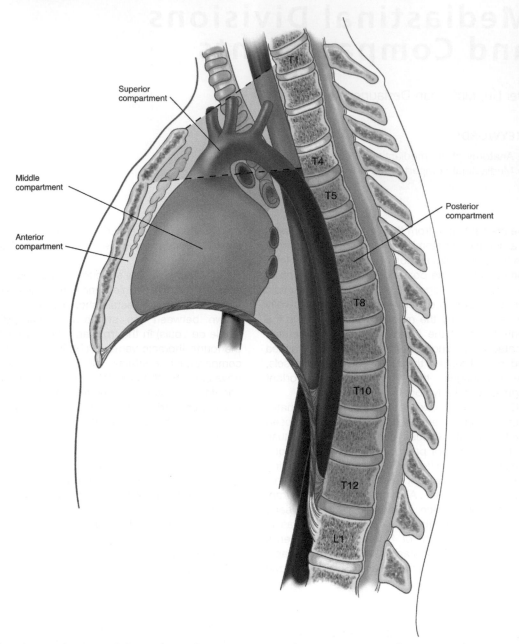

Fig. 1. Anatomic location of the mediastinal compartments in the 4-compartment scheme. Note the virtual line that separates the superior and inferior compartments.

Table 1
Boundaries and contents of the 4-compartment scheme

	Boundaries	Contents
Superior mediastinum	Thoracic inlet to line drawn from angle of Louis to T4	Aorta and great vessels, trachea, upper third of esophagus, upper thymus
Anterior mediastinum	Anterior to pericardium and posterior to body of sternum	Mediastinal fat and thymus
Middle mediastinum	Bounded anteriorly and posteriorly by pericardium	Pericardium and contents, carina, lymph nodes
Posterior mediastinum	Dorsal surface of pericardium to anterior surfaces of T1-T12	Esophagus, descending thoracic aorta, azygos vein, thoracic duct

contains the esophagus, descending thoracic aorta, azygos vein, thoracic duct, and sympathetic chains.

Three-Compartment Model

A popular modification of the 4-compartment scheme divides the mediastinum into 3 compartments (**Fig. 2**; **Table 2**): anterior (anterosuperior), middle, and posterior. This model does not recognize a specific superior mediastinal compartment.[4,5]

The anterior mediastinum extends from the thoracic inlet superiorly to the diaphragm inferiorly. It is bounded in the front by the posterior sternal

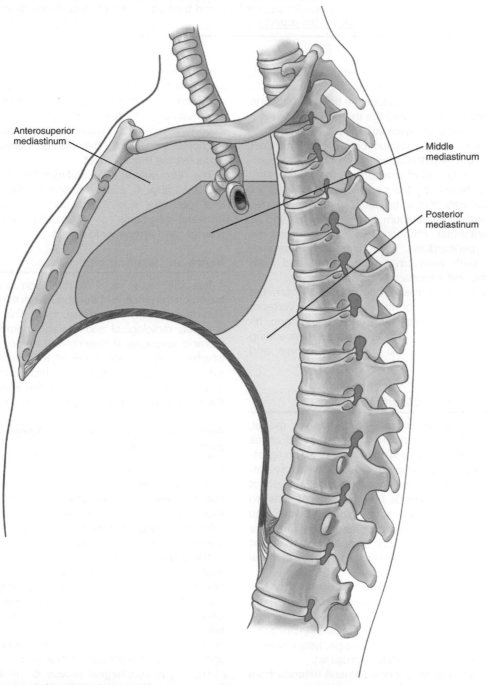

Fig. 2. Anatomic location of the mediastinal compartments in the 3-compartment model. In this model, there is no specific superior compartment.

Table 2
Boundaries and contents of the 3-compartment model

	Boundaries	Contents
Anterior mediastinum (antero-superior)	From thoracic inlet to diaphragm and from posterior sternum to pericardium	Adipose and mesenchymal tissues, thymus
Middle mediastinum	From anterior pericardium to posterior pericardium and posterior trachea	Heart, pericardium, aorta, main bronchi, lymph nodes
Posterior mediastinum	From posterior pericardium and trachea to ventral aspect of spine	Esophagus, descending aorta, vagus nerves, lymph nodes

table and in the back by the anterior pericardium, innominate vein, aorta, and brachiocephalic vessels. Its contents include the thymus, fatty and connective tissues, and the thyroid gland when it extends below the neck into the mediastinum.

The middle mediastinum contains all structures located between the anterior and posterior mediastinum. It is bounded anteriorly by the pericardium, and posteriorly by the pericardium and posterior tracheal wall. It is to be noted that in this model, the middle mediastinum extends only as high as the pericardial reflection. This space contains the heart, pericardium, ascending and transverse aorta, both vena cavae, the trachea and main bronchi, and important lymphatic channels.

The posterior mediastinum extends from the superior aspects of the first thoracic vertebra (thoracic inlet) inferiorly to the diaphragm. Its contents include the esophagus, descending thoracic aorta, thoracic duct, vagus nerves, and lymph nodes.

Shields' 3-Zone Classification

In 1972, Shields[2] suggested a different model, whereby the mediastinum is divided into 3 zones (**Fig. 3**; **Table 3**) consisting of an anterior compartment, a visceral compartment, and the paravertebral sulci (retrovisceral zone) bilaterally. Each of these 3 zones extends from the thoracic inlet to the diaphragm, and at the thoracic inlet, the visceral compartment occupies the entire space anterior to the spine. Each compartment is limited laterally by the mediastinal surfaces of their respective mediastinal pleura.

The most anterior compartment or prevascular zone extends from the undersurface of the sternum to the pericardium and anterior surfaces of the great vessels posteriorly. Its contents include the thymus, internal mammary vessels, lymph nodes, connective tissues, and pericardial fat.

The visceral zone (compartment) extends from the anterior reflection of the pericardium to the spinal anterior longitudinal ligament posteriorly

(anterior surface of the vertebral bodies). In this zone are the pericardium and its contents; the aortic arch and its branches; the trachea, carina, and main bronchi; the esophagus; and the most important lymphatic channels of the mediastinum. As noted by Shields, the visceral compartment occupies the thoracic inlet.

The retrovisceral zone includes the paravertebral sulci (**Fig. 4**), costovertebral junctions, proximal posterior ribs (head and neck of ribs), proximal segments of intercostal nerves and arteries, and sympathetic trunks.

Heitzman Classification

A less commonly used classification is the one based on the location of the aortic arch and azygos vein described in 1997 by Heitzman.[6] This scheme is purely radiological and is very impractical for thoracic surgeons. It describes 6 compartments, which consist of the thoracic inlet, the anterior mediastinum, the superior aortic area (above the aortic arch), the infra-aortic area (below the aortic arch), the supra-azygos area, and the infra-azygos area.

Aortopulmonary Window and Azygo-Esophageal Recess

The aortopulmonary window and azygo-esophageal recess are not pure mediastinal compartments but they are important because they contain lymph node stations that can be affected by lung or esophageal cancers that may present as mediastinal masses.

The aortopulmonary window is a middle mediastinal space bounded superiorly by the inferior margin of the aortic arch (**Fig. 5**), inferiorly by the posterior wall of the ascending aorta, and medially by the left main bronchus and esophagus.[4] It contains the left vagus and left recurrent laryngeal nerve. Approximately one-third of lung cancers located in the left upper lobe will metastasize in that area.

The azygo-esophageal recess is the interface between the right lung and the mediastinal reflection inferior to the arch of the azygos vein, with the

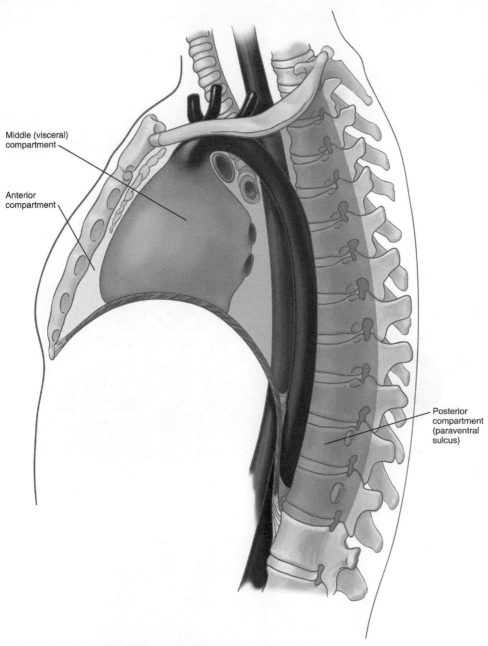

Middle (visceral) compartment

Anterior compartment

Posterior compartment (paraventral sulcus)

Fig. 3. Anatomic location of mediastinal compartments in Shields' 3-zone classification. In this model, each zone extends from the thoracic inlet to the diaphragm.

Table 3
Boundaries and contents of Shields' 3-zone classification

	Boundaries	Contents
Previsceral zone (anterior)	Under surface of sternum to anterior surface of pericardium and great vessels	Thymus, internal mammary vessels
Visceral zone	Anterior reflection of pericardium to anterior surface to spine	Pericardium and contents, trachea and main bronchi, esophagus
Retrovisceral zone	Paravertebral sulci	Costovertebral junctions, proximal intercostal nerves and arteries, sympathetic trunks

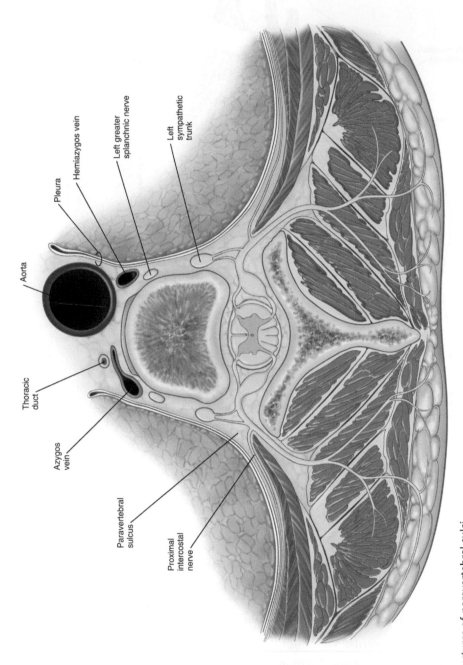

Fig. 4. Normal structures of paravertebral sulci.

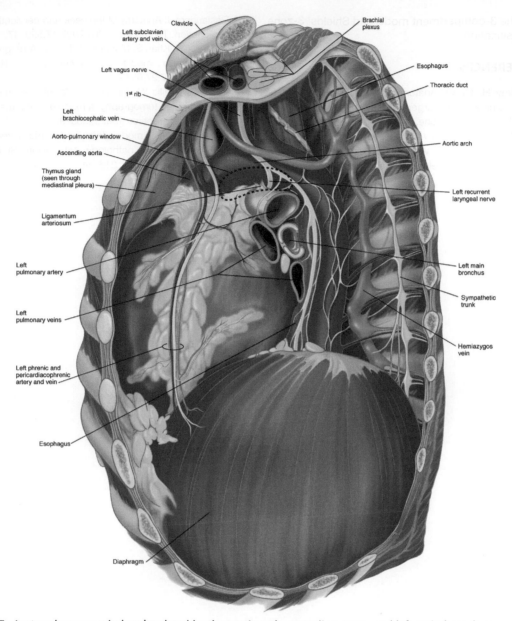

Fig. 5. Aortopulmonary window bordered by the aortic arch, ascending aorta, and left main bronchus.

esophagus lying anteriorly and the azygos vein posteriorly. Nodal enlargement in that area is often secondary to metastatic disease from esophageal carcinomas.

SUMMARY

Although it is practical to use mediastinal compartments to subdivide the mediastinum and classify mediastinal abnormalities, one has to remember that there are no real anatomic boundaries between the various mediastinal compartments and that tumors traditionally described in one compartment are not excluded from surrounding compartments. Indeed, diseases or tumors of the mediastinum often spread or extend from one compartment to another.

Having a clear understanding of the divisions of the mediastinum is nevertheless important for the thoracic surgeon who daily has to establish a differential diagnosis of mediastinal masses based on their location, as well as to select the best surgical approach to access the mediastinum to obtain diagnostic material, to drain mediastinal spaces, or to excise mediastinal tumors. In this respect, the most useful classifications appear to be the 3-compartment model and Shields' 3-zone classification.

REFERENCES

1. Gray H. Gray's Anatomy: The anatomical basis of medicine and surgery. 38th edition. New York: Churchill Livingstone; 1995.
2. Shields TW. Primary tumors and cysts of the mediastinum. In: Shields TW, editor. General thoracic surgery. 1st edition. Philadelphia: Lea and Febiger; 1972. p. 908.
3. Deslauriers J. Anatomy of the neck and cervicothoracic junction. Thorac Surg Clin 2007;17:529–47.
4. Whitten CR, Khan S, Munneke GJ, et al. A diagnostic approach to mediastinal abnormalities. Radiographics 2007;27:657–71.
5. Zylak CJ, Paillic W, Jackson R. Correlative anatomy and computed tomography: a module on the mediastinum. Radiographics 1982;2:555–92.
6. Heitzman ER. The mediastinum: radiologic correlation with anatomy and pathology. 1st edition. St Louis (MO): Mosby; 1977. p. 216–34.

Anatomy of the Thymus Gland

Najib Safieddine, MD, FRCSC[a],
Shaf Keshavjee, MD, MSc, FRCSC[b],*

KEYWORDS

• Thymus gland • Development • Anatomy • Blood supply

"Walking like smoke in the breasts if men even as Agamenon angered me, but we will let bygones be bygones quieting the thymos in our breasts"

Achilles, The Iliad

The early historical recognition of the thymus as a distinct structure contrasts with the much more recent recognition of its function.[1–5] Thought to be derived from the Greek word "thymos," which denotes life force, rise into flames, the function of the thymus gland remained illusive until the development of the science of immunology. It is also believed that Galen gave it the name thymus, because it reminded him of a bunch of thyme, burnt as incense for the Greek gods. If the ancient Greek notion of life force sounds more appropriate for the Iliad than a treatise of science, as late as the early 1900s, theories about the association of the thymus with feminism and sudden death remained almost as unsatisfactory to explain the enigmatic function. The historical association of the thymus with sudden death and so-called "status lymphaticus" is also very interesting. In the 17th and 18th centuries, many reported cases of sudden death believed to be associated with an enlarged thymus ultimately led to the theory of status lymphaticus (SL) in the 19th century. Introduced by Paltauf, SL was a syndrome believed to terminate (but not always) in sudden death secondary to enlarged thymus crushing the trachea or the vagus nerves. In the 1890s, sudden death was believed to be but one of the characteristics of SL, where lowered immunity to infection was now thought to be another important aspect.

It is not clear when the first thymectomy was performed, but McLennan in 1914 reported on 8 cases. Friedlander later reported 33% mortality. Collins in 1685, however, did speak of a physiologic connection between the thymus, lymph nodes, and tonsils, postulating that it received a "thin spirituous liquor" from the nerves and then attenuated it to pass it on to the general circulation.

DEVELOPMENT OF THE THYMUS GLAND

The thymus arises from the endoderm of the third and possibly fourth branchial pouches during the sixth week of gestation. During the seventh and eighth gestational weeks, the thymuses elongate and enlarge caudally and anterolaterally, culminating in the fusion of the advancing distal ends at the level of the of the superior margin of the aortic arch and the loss of its connection with the branchial clefts at the end of the eighth gestational week. Only connective tissue is affected by the fusion so that the glandular tissues of both lobes remain distinct. At the end of fusion, the thymus enlarges and attaches to the pericardium. This determines the permanent position of the gland in the anterior superior mediastinum. There is preferential enlargement of the caudal poles that ultimately become thicker than the cranial poles. The connections to the pharynx disappear at the end of the eighth gestational week, but islands of

[a] Division of Thoracic Surgery, Toronto General Hospital, University of Toronto, 200 Elizabeth Street 9N-946, Toronto, ON M5G 2G4, Canada
[b] Division of Thoracic Surgery, Toronto General Hospital, University Health Network, University of Toronto, 200 Elizabeth Street 9N-946, Toronto, ON M5G 2G4, Canada
* Corresponding author.
E-mail address: shaf.keshavjee@uhn.on.ca

Thorac Surg Clin 21 (2011) 191–195
doi:10.1016/j.thorsurg.2010.12.011

thymic tissue can be found in the tympanic cavity, neck, mediastinum, or lung. This occurs in 20% to 25% of people.

The thymus achieves its greatest weight proportional to body weight at birth and greatest absolute weight at puberty. Physiologic involution, a normal process, occurs with increased age and is associated parenchymal loss and fat replacement. This is a distinct process from early rapid or "accidental" involution mediated by increased corticosteroid levels.

GROSS ANATOMY

Anatomically, the earliest preserved drawings of the gland were the line drawings of Vesalius. Bertolini in 1684 gave a very lucid description of the gland with drawings. The thymus is located in the midline and generally lies in the anterior superior mediastinum (**Fig. 1**). It is a pinkish gray gland in color with a lobulated surface (**Fig. 2**). At birth it weighs approximately 13 g to 15 g and 35 g to 45 g at puberty. With onset of involution, its weight decreases to 25 g at 25 years and then further to less than 15 g at 60 years and 6 g at 70 years on average. The normal gland is about 5 cm in length, 4 cm in breadth, and 6 mm in thickness. Its surface landmarks are the inferior border of the thyroid gland superiorly, and the fourth intercostal cartilage inferiorly; it is bordered only by the sternum anteriorly.

The thymus is composed of two lobes slightly different in size, usually with a slightly larger right lobe. The two lobes are connected by loose connective tissue at the midline and occasionally by an intermediate lobe. It is enclosed by a sheath of connective fibrous tissue layer, forming a capsule that septates the gland, dividing each lobe into several lobules. The septa extend only as far as the corticomedullary junction, so that the medulla is confluent through out.

Superiorly, the thymus is often connected to the thyroid gland by the thyrothymic ligament, made of thin strands of connective tissue that contains minute blood vessels. Anteriorly, the thymus lies immediately behind the origins of the sternothyroid and the sternohyoid muscles in its cervical portions and the sternum in its mediastinal portions. Posteriorly, it lies immediately anterior to the brachiocephalic vein and aortic arch and its branches, to which it is connected by a layer of fascia. Inferiorly, the lower poles rest on the pericardium and are connected to it by thin strands of connective tissue. Laterally, the thymus runs along side the pleura and in close proximity to mediastinal fat and the phrenic nerves.

ARTERIAL SUPPLY

Although the thymus draws its blood supply from numerous branches of all arteries in its vicinity, three principle sources can be identified. The superior thymic arteries most commonly originate from the inferior thyroid artery (**Fig. 3**). Occasionally, they may arise from the middle thyroid artery. Laterally, the lateral thymic arteries are usually asymmetrical and variable in number. They originate from the internal mammary artery, more numerous on the right. Occasionally they arise from the superior phrenic artery (itself a branch of the internal mammary artery). The posterior thymic arteries are direct branches of the brachiocephalic artery and aorta, most commonly in the form of a single branch that divides into branches to both lobes before entering the capsule. Anomalous arterial supply has been reported from the internal carotid artery.

VENOUS DRAINAGE

The venous draining system of the thymus gland does not run parallel to its arterial supply. It commonly consists of larger veins that follow the interlobar septa into the thymic capsule and small veins that leave the cortex to form venous plexus on the posterior surface of the thymic capsule. The thymic posterior veins (grand veins of Keynes) are formed by the fusion of numerous smaller veins that drain the gland and in turn empty into the brachiocephalic vein just proximal to the origin

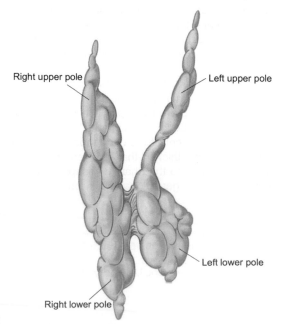

Right upper pole

Left upper pole

Left lower pole

Right lower pole

Fig. 1. The thymus gland.

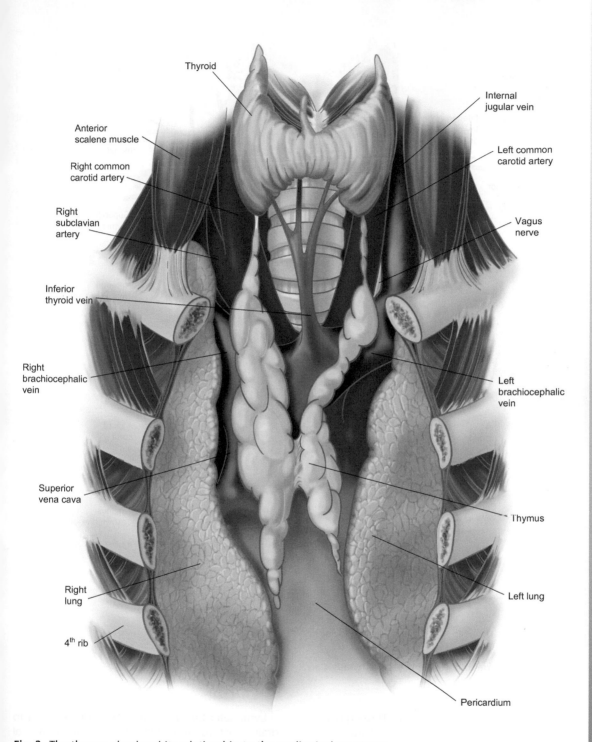

Fig. 2. The thymus gland and its relationship to the mediastinal structures.

of the superior intercostal vein (**Fig. 4**). Superior thymic veins drain the superior aspect of the gland in 50% of cases and empty into the inferior thyroid vein. Other rarer, smaller, and less consistent veins drain into the superior vena cava, thyriodea IMA (internal mammary vein).

LYMPHATIC VESSELS

No afferent lymphatic system is known to enter the thymus. Small lymphatic capillaries originating in the perivascular spaces of the medulla converge to form larger vessels that run along perilobular

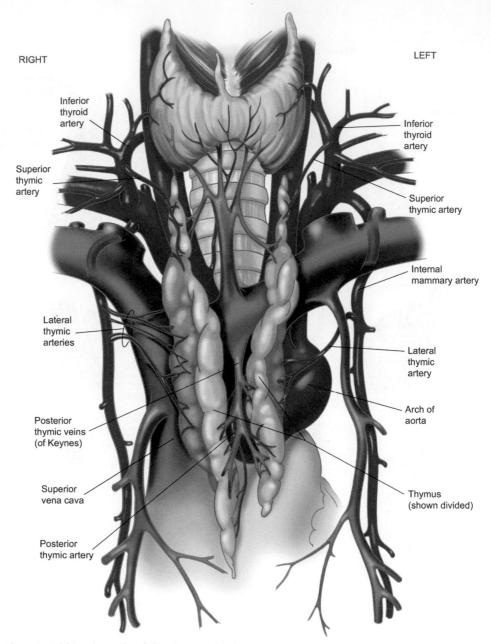

RIGHT

LEFT

Inferior thyroid artery

Inferior thyroid artery

Superior thymic artery

Superior thymic artery

Internal mammary artery

Lateral thymic arteries

Lateral thymic artery

Posterior thymic veins (of Keynes)

Arch of aorta

Superior vena cava

Thymus (shown divided)

Posterior thymic artery

Fig. 3. The arterial blood supply of the thymus gland.

veins to the level of the capsule. Three groups of lymphatic drainage have been identified:

1. The superior lymphatic ducts draining the caudal portions into the internal jugular, innominate, or anterior mediastinal nodes
2. The more numerous anterior lymphatic ducts that drain into the parasternal lymph nodes
3. The posterior lymphatic ducts that drain into the tracheobronchial lymph nodes.

Lymphatic basins (2) and (3) ultimately join to drain most commonly into the ipsilateral internal jugular and subclavian veins.

INNERVATION OF THE THYMUS

The innervation of the thymus is numerous and variable and generally nondistinct. The descending vagus, phrenic, hypoglossal, and occasionally the recurrent laryngeal nerves all contribute branches to the thymus.

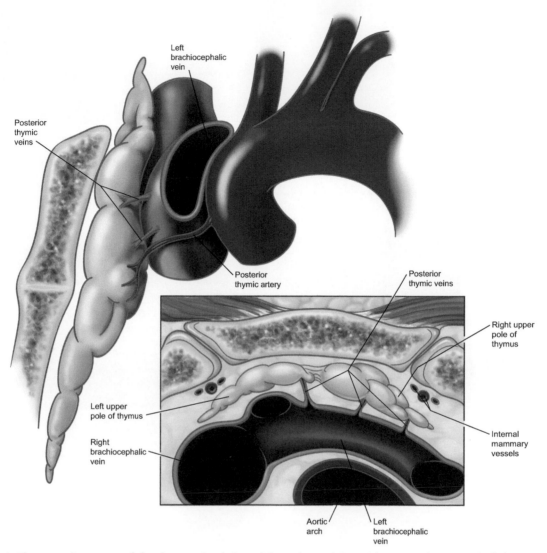

Fig. 4. The posterior aspect of the thymus gland viewed from the neck in a video-assisted transcervical thymectomy illustrating two thymic veins draining into the innominate vein.

SUMMARY

In the case of the thymus gland, the most common indications for resection are myasthenia gravis or thymoma. In any form of surgery, thorough knowledge of the anatomy is the key to a safe and effective operation. The consistency and appearance of the thymus gland make it difficult at times to discern from mediastinal fatty tissues. The nature of the embryologic development and variations in the size and shape of the gland from patient to patient and with age make definition of the anatomic features even more challenging. Therefore having a clear understanding of the anatomy and the relationship of the gland to adjacent structures is important.

REFERENCES

1. Goss JA, Flye MW. The thymus—regulator of cellular immunity. In: Medical intelligence unit. Austin (TX): R.G. Landes Co; 1993.
2. Cardarelli NF. Role of the thymus in health and senescence: thymus and immunity. Boca Raton (FL): CRC Press; 1989.
3. Netter FH, Dalley AF. Atlas of human anatomy. 2nd edition. New York (NY): Novartis; 1997.
4. Henry K, Farrer-Brown G. A color atlas of thymus and lymph node histopathology: with ultrastructure. Prescott (AZ): Wolfe; 1981.
5. Gray H. Gray's anatomy: the anatomical basis of clinical practice. Livingston; 2005. p. 1825–61.

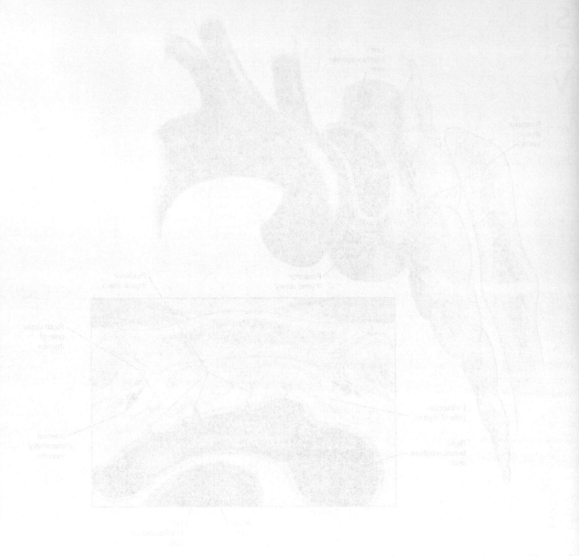

Anatomy of the Superior Vena Cava and Brachiocephalic Veins

W. Frederick Bennett, BSc, MD, FRCS(C)[a],
Fawaz Altaf, MB, ChB, FRCS(C), FRCS(I)[a],
Jean Deslauriers, MD, FRCS(C)[b],*

KEYWORDS
• Superior vena cava • Brachiocephalic veins • Anatomy
• Pneumonectomy

ANATOMY OF THE SUPERIOR VENA CAVA AND BRACHIOCEPHALIC VEINS

The venous side of the systemic vascular circulation returns the left ventricular cardiac output in a converging fashion to the superior and inferior vena cava and hence to the right atrium.[1–4] The volumes of these 2 systems are in balance in a normal physiologic state. Cephalad to the diaphragm, the mediastinal and superficial systems coalesce integrating virtually all of the systemic venous return to the right atrium through the superior vena cava (**Tables 1** and **2**).

The exceptions to this normal state include the return of the coronary arterial blood flow via the coronary sinus to the right atrium and via the thebesian veins to the ventricular chambers, as well as bronchial venous flow distal to the third division of the bronchial tree bilaterally, which returns along with the oxygenated blood in the pulmonary venous system to the left atrium (see **Table 1**).

In the performance of pulmonary resections, the systemic veins are not of frequent concern. However, in the surgical treatment of mediastinal disease they are of more pivotal importance.

EMBRYOLOGY

The systemic and cardiopulmonary vessels form in the human embryo during the first 3 to 8 weeks of gestation at the 2- to 37-mm stage of development. The process is extremely complex as ontogeny recapitulates phylogeny. Genetic control, induction, collision, rotation, and folding of the vascular structures combine to form the cardiopulmonary system, which (apart from closure of fetal bypass circulation at parturition), is essentially complete during the first trimester of pregnancy.

The right venous horn enlarges with increasing volume of flow and the right superior vena cava is formed from the proximal right anterior cardinal vein, and the right brachiocephalic vein arises from the distal analog. As drainage of the venous horn decreases secondary to obliteration of its upper and lower cardinal veins, the remnant forms the coronary sinus and the oblique vein of Marshal, which is connected superiorly to the fibrous remains of the left superior vena cava (**Fig. 1**). Both of these structures are incorporated in a triangular fold of serous pericardium, named the vestigial fold of Marshal, extending cephalad to the left

[a] Division of Thoracic Surgery, Department of Surgery, McMaster University, St Joseph's Healthcare, Juravinski Innovation Tower, 2nd Floor, Room T2105J, 50 Charlton Avenue East, Hamilton, Ontario L8N 4A6, Canada
[b] Institut Universitaire de Cardiologie et de Pneumologie de Québec, Laval University, 2725 Chemin Sainte-Foy, Quebec City, Quebec G1V 4G5, Canada
* Corresponding author.
E-mail address: Jean.Deslauriers@fmed.ulaval.ca

Thorac Surg Clin 21 (2011) 197–203
doi:10.1016/j.thorsurg.2010.12.010
1547-4127/11/$ – see front matter © 2011 Published by Elsevier Inc.

Table 1
Systemic venous return bypassing the superior vena cava

Coronary veins entering the coronary sinus in the right atrium

Coronary venous return to the right and left ventricle via the thebesian veins

Bronchial venous drainage distal to third generation of bronchial tree entering the pulmonary venous system to the left atrium

superior intercostal vein. On rare occasion, this vein may be patent and pose a hazard during intrapericardial left pneumonectomy.

THE BRACHIOCEPHALIC VEINS
Right Brachiocephalic Vein

The right brachiocephalic vein begins at the confluence of the right internal jugular and right subclavian veins posterior to the sternal end of the clavicle and anterior to the pleura and vagus nerve. It descends for 2 to 3 cm to the point where the pleura, right phrenic nerve, and internal thoracic artery and vein form its lateral relationship. The thymus gland and brachiocephalic artery are juxtaposed medially. This vessel joins the left brachiocephalic vein at the level of the lower border of the first right costal cartilage to become the superior vena cava.

Tributaries to the right brachiocephalic vein include the right vertebral vein joining it superiorly and the internal thoracic veins doing so laterally.

Table 2
Points of interest

The space between the posterior wall of the superior vena cava and the anterior right main pulmonary artery must be free to allow proximal control of the latter structure during a right pneumonectomy.

The vestigial vein of Marshall may be patent in the pericardial fold over the left intrapericardial pulmonary artery mandating control during an intrapericardial left pneumonectomy.

The azygous vein can be falsely cannulated with resultant injury during institution of cardiopulmonary bypass.

Intraoperative detection of a venous abnormality should alert the surgeon to the probability that other anomalies of the systemic and pulmonary circulation and the bronchial tree may be encountered during a thoracic surgical procedure.

Further tributaries consist of the anterior mediastinal veins, the pericardial veins, the sternal veins, and the anterior intercostal veins of the upper 6 intercostal spaces. Occasionally the right superior intercostal vein integrating the first to fourth intercostal veins drains to it directly instead of to the azygos system. The inferior thyroid vein also enters it medially.

Left Brachiocephalic Vein

This structure is longer than its contralateral equivalent and runs for about 6 cm in length beginning behind the sternal end of the left clavicle and progressing obliquely downward and to the right behind the manubrium sterni of the right first costal cartilage of the right first rib where it unites with the right vein (**Fig. 2**). Its posterior relationships include the innominate artery, left common carotid artery, and left subclavian artery together with the vagus and phrenic nerves.

Its tributaries are the same as the right-sided analog with the addition of the left superior intercostal vein draining the upper 3 or 4 intercostal spaces as well as a variable number of inferior thymic veins entering its superior aspect. Pericardial tributaries also interface with this structure.

Superior Vena Cava

From the junction of the 2 brachiochephalic veins, the superior vena cava formed by the confluence of these two veins passes caudal and proceeds approximately 7 cm joining the superior aspect of the right atrium posterior to the upper border of the right third costal cartilage. Its distal portion is enveloped by the pericardium. The phrenic nerve has a direct lateral relationship to this structure and its medial relationships include the innominate artery and the ascending aorta. The final tributary to the superior vena cava near its termination is the azygos vein passing over the upper aspect of the right main stem bronchus from its posterior course (**Figs. 3** and **4**).

This structure originates from calescence of the right subcostal and intercostal veins on the right and the hemiazygos vein, which pass from the left anterior to the spinal column. Several esophageal, mediastinal, and pericardial veins contribute to this vessel and the bronchial veins draining the first 3 divisions of the bronchial tree represent rather minor tributaries. The tissue plane between the posterior wall of the distal superior vena cava and the anterior wall of the right main pulmonary artery is referred to surgically as the retro caval space of Allison and is of particular significance in the performance of both standard and extended right pneumonectomies.

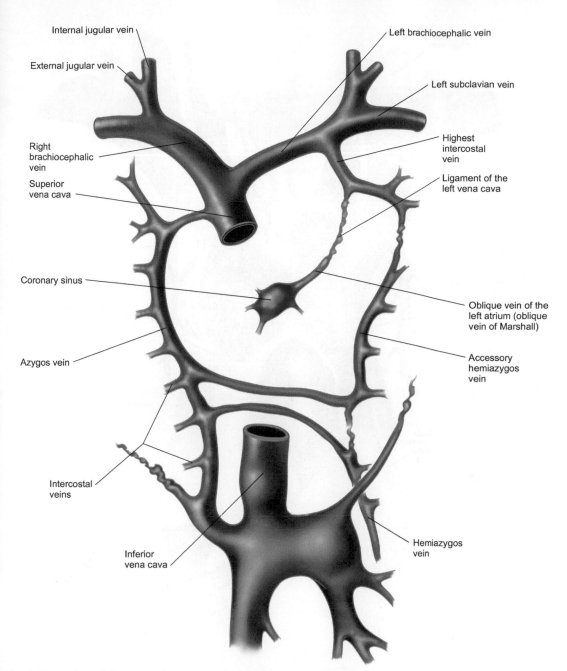

Fig. 1. Formation of the systemic venous system in the embryo. Note the oblique vein of Marshall which is connected to the fibrous remnant of the left superior vena cava. (ligament of left vena cava).

Mediastinal Veins and the Thoracic Surgeon

Surgical management of the systemic veins of the thorax is largely a matter of avoidance of injury to these structures (see **Table 2**). The venous drainage of the thymus gland is discussed in another section

by Safieddine and Keshavjee of this issue. In terms of pulmonary resections, the azygos vein is often ligated to facilitate exposure of the origin of the right main bronchus and carina. Rarely, the azygos vein creates a fissure within the right upper lobe and this medial segment will lie central to the mediastinal

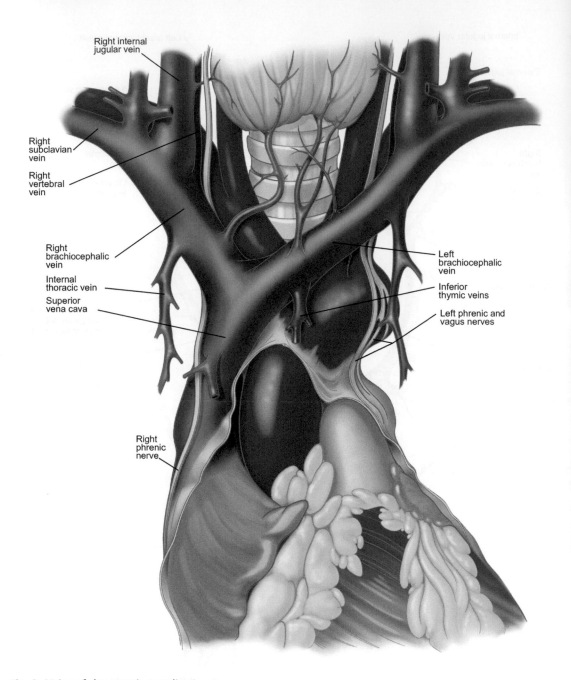

Fig. 2. Veins of the superior mediastinum.

Labels on figure:
Right internal jugular vein
Right subclavian vein
Right vertebral vein
Right brachiocephalic vein
Internal thoracic vein
Superior vena cava
Right phrenic nerve
Left brachiocephalic vein
Inferior thymic veins
Left phrenic and vagus nerves

pleura above the vein. The left superior intercostal vein generally requires division to perform a supra-aortic left pneumonectomy.

Several congenital venous anomalies are diagnosed and treated in the neonatal and childhood age group by pediatric general and cardiac surgeons. However, the preoperative or intraoperative finding of a systemic venous abnormality should always alert the thoracic surgeon operating on adult patients. The probability of additional systemic and pulmonary circulatory anomalies as well as those of the bronchial tree is significantly increased in these situations and due caution should be exercised intraoperatively.

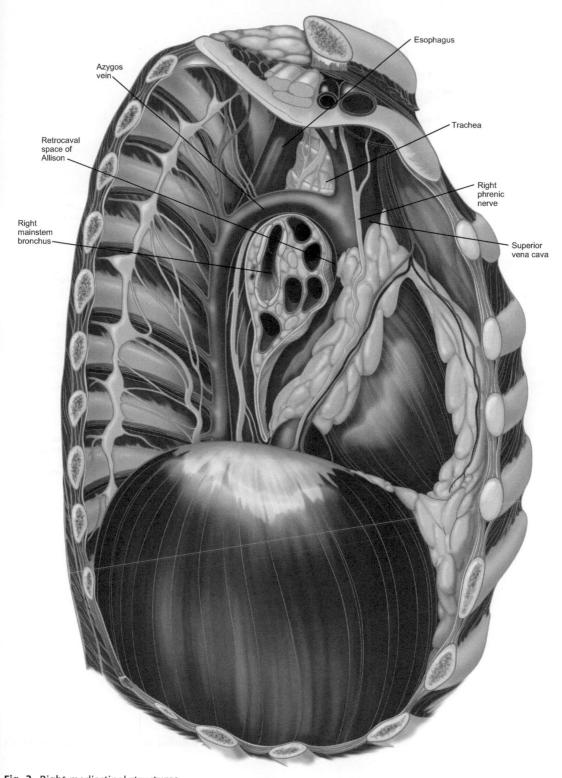

Fig. 3. Right mediastinal structures.

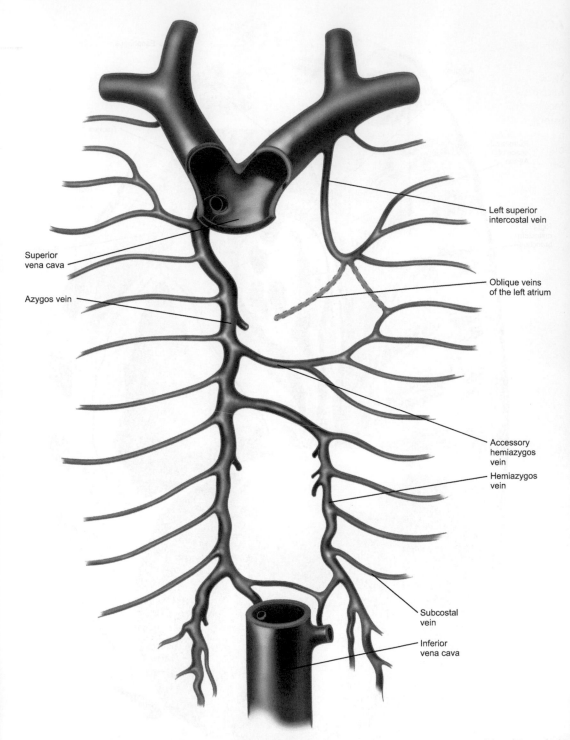

Fig. 4. Azygos, hemiazygos, and posterior intercostals tributaries to the superior vena cava and brachiocephalic veins.

ACKNOWLEDGMENTS

The author expresses his gratitude to R. Abbey Smith, formerly Consultant Thoracic Surgeon, Walsgrave Hospital, Coventry, and to the West Midlands Regional Health Authority UK for many technical surgical anatomy lessons, including intraoperative recognition and management of a persistent vein of Marshall during an intrapericardial left pneumonectomy. His teachings have served my patients well.

REFERENCES

1. Langman J. Medical embryology. 6th edition. Baltimore (MA): Williams and Wilkins; 1990.
2. Jones KL. Smith's recognizable patterns of human malformation. Philadelphia (PA): W.B. Saunders; 1997.
3. Agur AMR, Dalley AF. Grant's atlas of anatomy. 11th edition. Baltimore (MA): Lippincott Williams & Wilkins; 2005.
4. Collis JL, Clarke DB, Abbey SR. D'Abreu's practice of cardiothoracic surgery. 4th edition. London: Edward Arnold Ltd; 1976.

ACKNOWLEDGMENTS

The author expresses his gratitude to R. Abbey Smith, formerly Consultant Thoracic Surgeon, Walsgrave Hospital, Coventry, and to the West Midlands Regional Health Authority UK for many technical surgical anatomy lessons, including intraoperative recognition and management of persistent left Marshall during an inappropriate, dificult left pneumonectomy. His teachings have served my patients well.

REFERENCES

1. Langman J. Medical embryology. 3rd edition. Baltimore (MA): Williams and Wilkins; 1963.
2. Moore KL. Smith's recognizable patterns of human malformation. Philadelphia (PA): W.B. Saunders; 1997.
3. Agur AMR, Dalley AF. Grant's atlas of anatomy. 11th edition. Baltimore (MA): Lippincott Williams & Wilkins; 2005.
4. Collis JL, Clarke DB, Abbey SR. D'Abreu's practical cardiothoracic surgery. 4th edition. London: Edward Arnold Ltd; 1976.

The Heart and Pericardium

Shahab A. Akhter, MD

KEYWORDS

• Heart • Pericardium • Anatomy • Cardiothoracic surgery

This article describes the normal anatomy of the heart and pericardium. Included is a detailed description of the pericardium, mediastinal nerves, cardiac chambers, valves, coronary arteries and veins, and the conduction tissues. A thorough knowledge of the anatomy of these structures is essential for the cardiothoracic surgeon.

THE PERICARDIUM

The heart lies within the pericardium, which is attached to the walls of the great vessels and to the diaphragm (**Fig. 1**). The inner layer, the visceral pericardium, is in direct contact with the heart. The outer layer forms the parietal pericardium, which lines the surface of the fibrous pericardial sack. A thin layer of fluid lies within the pericardial cavity between the 2 serous layers. Two recesses lie within the pericardium and are lined by the serous layer. The transverse sinus is delineated anteriorly by the posterior surface of the aorta and main pulmonary artery, and posteriorly by the anterior surface of the interatrial groove. The oblique sinus is a cul-de-sac located behind the left atrium, which is delineated by serous pericardial reflections from the pulmonary veins and the inferior vena cava.

The vagus and phrenic nerves descend through the mediastinum in close relationship to the heart. They enter through the thoracic inlet with the phrenic nerve located on the anterior surface of the anterior scalene muscle and posterior to the internal thoracic artery at the level of the thoracic inlet. On the right side, the phrenic nerve courses on the lateral surface of the superior vena cava. The nerve then descends anterior to the pulmonary hilum before reflecting onto the right diaphragm, where it branches to provide its

innervation. In the case of a left-sided superior caval vein, the left phrenic nerve is located on its lateral surface. The nerve passes anteriorly to the pulmonary hilum and eventually branches on the surface of the diaphragm. The vagus nerves enter the thorax posterior to the phrenic nerves and course along the carotid arteries. On the right, the vagus gives off the recurrent laryngeal nerve that passes around the right subclavian artery before ascending out of the thoracic cavity. The right vagus nerve continues posterior to the pulmonary hilum, gives off branches of the right pulmonary plexus, and exits the thorax along the esophagus. On the left, the vagus nerve crosses the aortic arch, where it gives off the recurrent laryngeal branch. The recurrent nerve passes around the ligamentum arteriosum before ascending in the tracheoesophageal groove. The vagus nerve continues posterior to the pulmonary hilum, gives rise to the left pulmonary plexus, and then continues inferiorly out of the thorax along the esophagus. A delicate nerve trunk, the subclavian loop, carries fibers from the stellate ganglion to the eye and head. This branch is located adjacent to the subclavian arteries bilaterally. Excessive dissection of the subclavian artery may lead to injury of these nerve roots and cause Horner syndrome.

CARDIAC CHAMBERS AND THE GREAT ARTERIES

The surgical anatomy of the heart is best understood when the position of the cardiac chambers and great vessels is known in relation to the cardiac silhouette (**Fig. 2**). The atrioventricular junction is oriented obliquely, lying much closer to the vertical than to the horizontal plane. This

Section of Cardiac and Thoracic Surgery, The University of Chicago, 5841 South Maryland Avenue, MC 5040, Chicago, IL 60637, USA
E-mail address: sakhter@surgery.bsd.uchicago.edu

Thorac Surg Clin 21 (2011) 205–217
doi:10.1016/j.thorsurg.2011.01.007

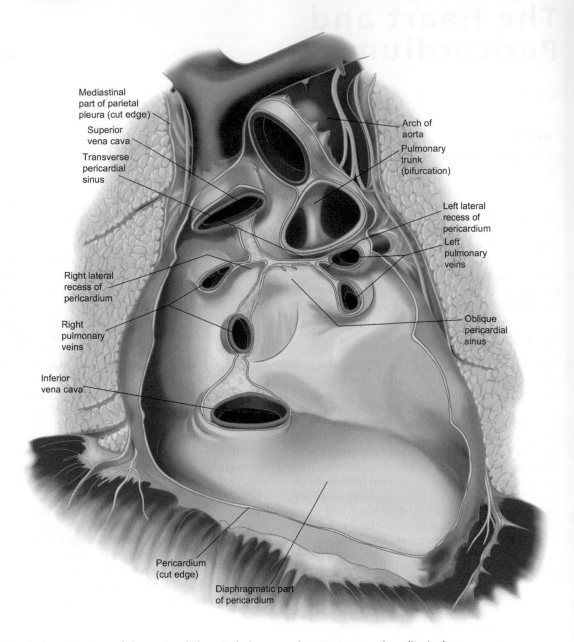

Mediastinal
part of parietal
pleura (cut edge)

Superior
vena cava

Transverse
pericardial
sinus

Arch of
aorta

Pulmonary
trunk
(bifurcation)

Left lateral
recess of
pericardium

Left
pulmonary
veins

Right lateral
recess of
pericardium

Right
pulmonary
veins

Oblique
pericardial
sinus

Inferior
vena cava

Pericardium
(cut edge)

Diaphragmatic part
of pericardium

Fig. 1. Anterior view of the pericardial sac including vascular structures and mediastinal nerves.

plane can be viewed from its atrial aspect if the atria and great arteries are removed by a parallel cut above the atrioventricular junction. The tricuspid and pulmonary valves are separated by the inner curvature of the heart lined by the transverse sinus. The mitral and aortic valves lie adjacent to one another, with fibrous continuity of their leaflets. The aortic valve occupies a central position, wedged between the tricuspid and pulmonary valves. There is also fibrous continuity between the leaflets of the aortic and tricuspid valves through the central fibrous body.

The atrial chambers lie to the right of their corresponding ventricles. The right atrium and ventricle lie anterior to the left atrium and ventricle. The septal structures between them are obliquely oriented. By virtue of its central position, the aortic valve is directly related to all of the cardiac chambers. The position of the aortic valve minimizes the area of septum where the mitral and tricuspid valves attach opposite each other. Because the tricuspid valve is attached to the septum further toward the ventricular apex than the mitral valve, a part of the septum is interposed between the

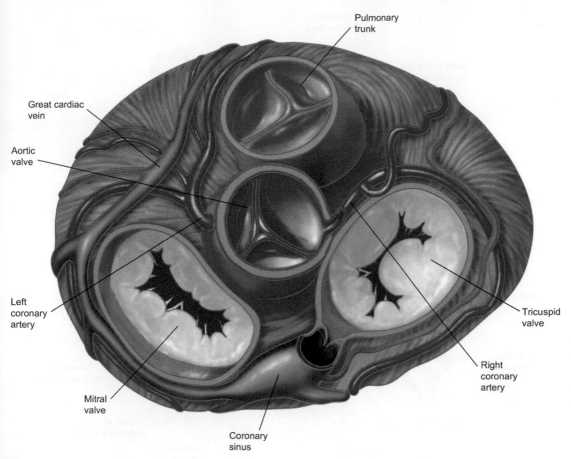

Pulmonary
trunk

Great cardiac
vein

Aortic
valve

Left
coronary
artery

Tricuspid
valve

Right
coronary
artery

Mitral
valve

Coronary
sinus

Fig. 2. Short-axis view of the heart. The atrioventricular junction is seen from above, having removed the atria and arterial trunks.

right atrium and the left ventricle to produce the muscular atrioventricular septum. The central fibrous body, where the leaflets of the aortic, mitral, and tricuspid valves all converge, lies cephalad and anterior to the muscular atrioventricular septum. The central fibrous body is the primary component of the fibrous skeleton of the heart and is made up, in part, by the right fibrous trigone, a thickening of the right side of the area of fibrous continuity between the aortic and mitral valves, and in part by the membranous septum, the fibrous partition between the left ventricular outflow tract and the right heart chambers. The membranous septum is divided into 2 parts by the septal leaflet of the tricuspid valve. Thus, the membranous septum has an atrioventricular component between the right atrium and left ventricle, as well as an interventricular portion.

THE RIGHT ATRIUM

The right atrium is divided into the appendage and the venous component, which receives the systemic venous return (**Fig. 3**). The junction of the appendage and the venous component is identified by a prominent groove known as the terminal groove, which corresponds internally to the location of the terminal crest. The most characteristic and constant feature of the morphology of the right atrium is that the pectinate muscles within the appendage extend around the entire parietal margin of the atrioventricular junction. These muscles originate as parallel fibers that course at right angles from the terminal crest. The venous component of the right atrium extends between the terminal groove and the interatrial groove. It receives blood from the superior and inferior caval veins and the coronary sinus.

The sinus node lies at the anterior and superior extent of the terminal groove, where the atrial appendage and the superior caval vein are adjoined. The node is a spindle-shaped structure that usually lies to the right or lateral to the superior cavoatrial junction. The blood supply to the sinus node is from a prominent nodal artery that is a branch of the right coronary artery in

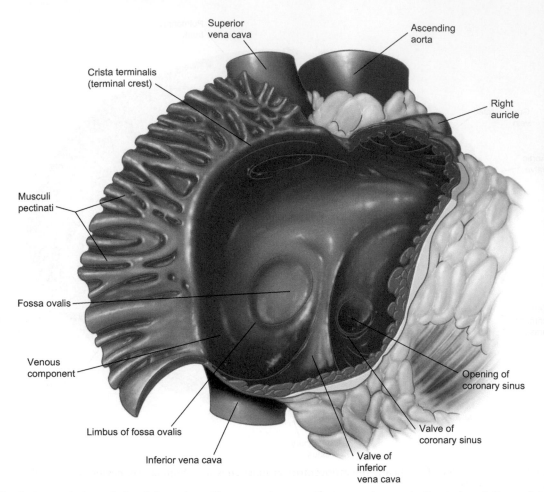

Superior
vena cava

Ascending
aorta

Crista terminalis
(terminal crest)

Right
auricle

Musculi
pectinati

Fossa ovalis

Venous
component

Opening of
coronary sinus

Limbus of fossa ovalis

Valve of
coronary sinus

Inferior vena cava

Valve of
inferior
vena cava

Fig. 3. Internal view of the right atrium. The appendage pectinate muscles create the trabeculations of the appendage in contrast with the smooth-walled venous component.

approximately 55% of individuals, and a branch of the left circumflex artery in the rest of the population. Regardless of its origin, the nodal artery usually courses along the anterior interatrial groove toward the superior cavoatrial junction, and frequently within the atrial myocardium. The artery may also arise distally from the circumflex artery and cross the dome of the left atrium.

In addition to the sinus node, another important component of the conduction system is the atrioventricular node. This structure lies within the triangle of Koch, which is demarcated by the tendon of Todaro, the septal leaflet of the tricuspid valve, and the orifice of the coronary sinus. The tendon of Todaro is a fibrous structure formed by the junction of the eustachian valve and the thebesian valve (the valves of the inferior caval vein and the coronary sinus, respectively). The entire atrial component of the atrioventricular conduction tissues is contained within the triangle of Koch. The atrioventricular bundle of His penetrates

directly at the apex of the triangle of Koch before it continues to branch on the crest of the ventricular septum.

THE TRICUSPID VALVE

The vestibule of the right atrium converges into the tricuspid valve (**Fig. 4**). The 3 leaflets reflect their anatomic location: septal, anterosuperior, and inferior. The leaflets are tethered at the commissures by fan-shaped cords arising from the papillary muscles. The anteroseptal commissure is supported by the medial papillary muscle. The major leaflets of the valve extend from this position in the anterosuperior and septal directions. The third leaflet is less well defined. The anteroinferior commissure is usually supported by the prominent anterior papillary muscle. It is often not possible to identify a specific inferior papillary muscle supporting the inferoseptal commissure. Thus, the inferior leaflet may appear duplicated. There is

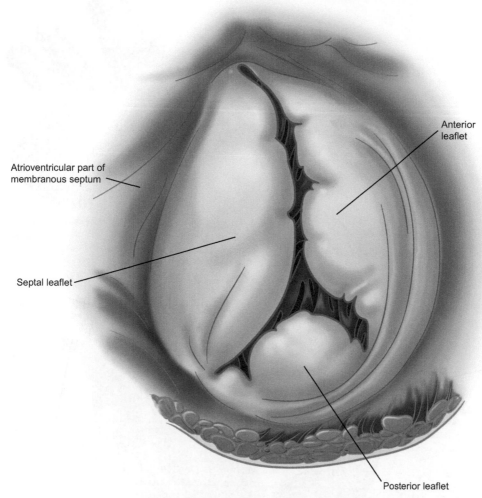

Anterior
leaflet

Atrioventricular part of
membranous septum

Septal leaflet

Posterior leaflet

Fig. 4. The tricuspid valve viewed from the right atrium at the atrioventricular junction. The position of the septal, anterosuperior, and inferior leaflets is shown.

no well-formed collagenous annulus for the tricuspid valve; rather, the atrioventricular groove folds directly into the tricuspid leaflets at the vestibule, and the atrium and ventricle are separated almost exclusively by the groove. The entire parietal attachment of the tricuspid valve usually is encircled by the right coronary artery running within the atrioventricular groove.

THE LEFT ATRIUM

The left atrium has 3 basic components: the appendage, vestibule, and venous components (**Fig. 5**). Unlike the right atrium, the venous component is larger than the appendage and has a narrow junction with it that is not marked by a terminal groove or crest. The left atrial appendage has a limited junction with the vestibule, and the pectinate muscles are located almost exclusively within the appendage. The larger part of the vestibule,

which supports and inserts directly into the posterior leaflet of the mitral valve, is directly continuous with the smooth atrial wall of the pulmonary venous component. The left atrium is posteriorly located and tethered by the 4 pulmonary veins.

THE MITRAL VALVE

The mitral valve is supported by 2 prominent papillary muscles located in anterolateral and posteromedial positions (**Fig. 6**). The 2 leaflets of the mitral valve are significantly different in appearance. The aortic (or anterior) leaflet is short, square, and covers approximately one-third of the circumference of the valvular orifice. This leaflet is in fibrous continuity with the aortic valve. The posterior leaflet is shallower but covers approximately two-thirds of the circumference of the mitral orifice. Because it is connected to the parietal portion of the atrioventricular junction, it is most

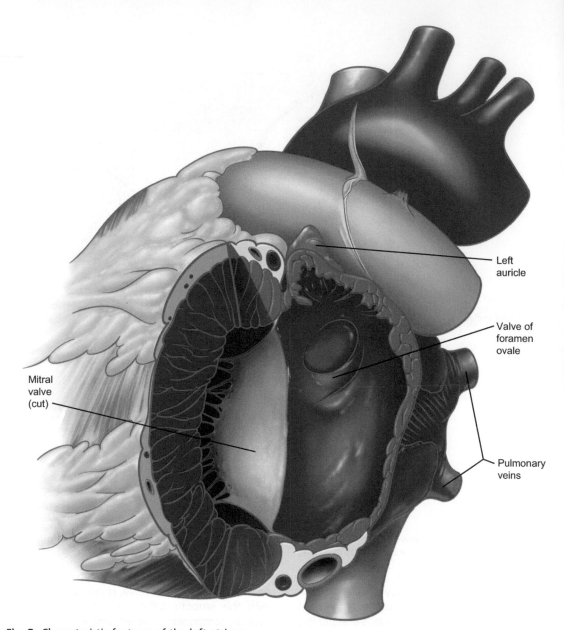

Left auricle

Valve of foramen ovale

Mitral valve (cut)

Pulmonary veins

Fig. 5. Characteristic features of the left atrium.

accurately named the mural leaflet, but is most commonly termed the posterior leaflet. It is typically divided into 3 segments that fold against the aortic leaflet when the valve is closed, named P1, P2, and P3. The mitral valve leaflets are supported by a dense collagenous annulus, although it may take the form of a sheet rather than a cord. This annulus usually extends parietally from the fibrous trigones, the thickened areas at either end of the area of fibrous continuity between the leaflets of the aortic and mitral valves. The midportion of the anterior leaflet of the mitral valve is related to the commissure between the noncoronary and left coronary cusps of the aortic valve.

The circumflex coronary artery is adjacent to the left half of the posterior leaflet, and the coronary sinus is adjacent to the right half of the posterior leaflet. When the circumflex artery is dominant, the entire attachment of the posterior leaflet may be intimately related to this artery.

THE RIGHT VENTRICLE AND PULMONARY VALVE

The inlet portion of the right ventricle surrounds the tricuspid valve and its chordal apparatus (**Fig. 7**). The apical trabecular portion of the right ventricle extends out to the apex. The outlet portion of the

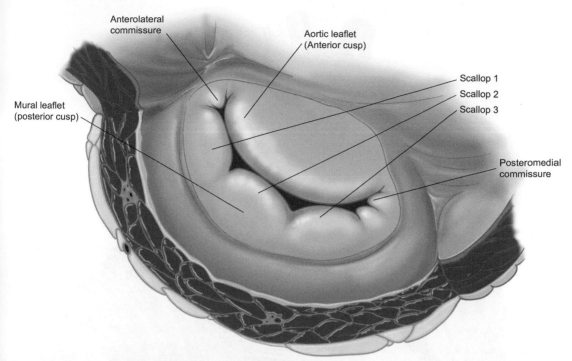

Anterolateral commissure

Aortic leaflet (Anterior cusp)

Scallop 1
Scallop 2
Scallop 3

Mural leaflet (posterior cusp)

Posteromedial commissure

Fig. 6. The atrial aspect of the mitral valve showing the anterior and posterior leaflets and commissures. The posterior leaflet has 3 segments or scallops: P1, P2, and P3.

right ventricle consists of the infundibulum, a circumferential muscular structure that supports the leaflets of the pulmonary valve. This valve does not have a traditional ringlike annulus because of the semilunar shape of the pulmonary valvar leaflets. The leaflets have semilunar attachments that cross the musculoarterial junction in a corresponding semilunar fashion. Therefore, instead of a single annulus, 3 rings can be distinguished anatomically in relation to the pulmonary valve. Superiorly, the sinotubular ridge of the pulmonary trunk marks the level of the commissures. A second ring exists at the ventriculoarterial junction, and a third ring can be constructed by joining the basal attachments of the 3 leaflets to the infundibular muscle.

A distinguishing feature of the right ventricle is a prominent muscular shelf, the supraventricular crest, which separates the tricuspid and pulmonary valves. This muscular ridge is the posterior part of the subpulmonary muscular infundibulum that supports the leaflets of the pulmonary valve. When the infundibulum is removed from the right ventricle, the insertion of the supraventricular crest between the limbs of the septomarginal trabeculation is visible. This trabeculation is a prominent muscle column that divides superiorly into anterior and posterior limbs. The anterior limb runs superiorly into the infundibulum and supports the leaflets of the pulmonary valve. The posterior limb extends

backward beneath the ventricular septum and runs into the inlet portion of the ventricle. The medial papillary muscle arises from this posterior limb. The body of the septomarginal trabeculation runs to the apex of the ventricle, where it divides into smaller trabeculations. Two of these trabeculations may be particularly prominent. One becomes the anterior papillary muscle and the other crosses the ventricular cavity as the moderator band.

THE LEFT VENTRICLE

Similar to the right ventricle, the left ventricle can be divided into 3 components (**Fig. 8**). The inlet component surrounds, and is limited by, the mitral valve and its chordal apparatus. The 2 papillary muscles occupy anterolateral and posteromedial positions and are positioned close to each other. The apical trabecular component of the left ventricle extends to the apex, where the myocardium is thin. The trabeculations of the left ventricle are fine compared with the right ventricle. The outlet component supports the aortic valve and consists of both muscular and fibrous portions, in contrast with the right ventricular infundibulum, which is composed entirely of muscle. The septal portion of the left ventricular outflow tract, although primarily muscular, also includes the

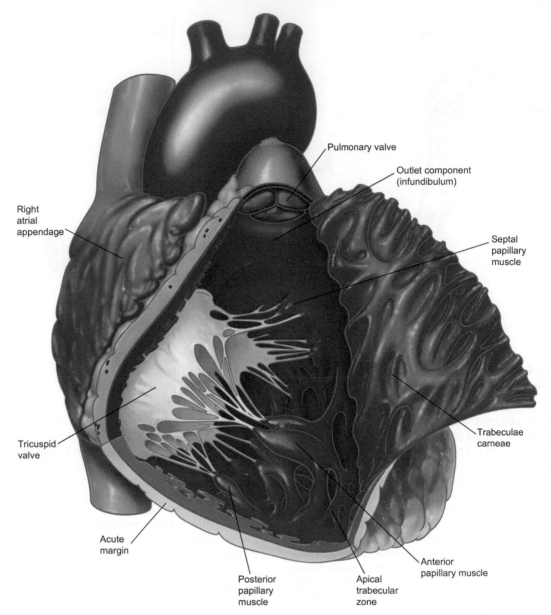

Fig. 7. The anterior wall of the right ventricle has been removed, showing the characteristic features of this chamber including the right ventricular outflow tract and the pulmonary valve.

membranous portion of the ventricular septum. The posterior quadrant of the outflow tract consists of an extensive fibrous curtain that extends from the fibrous skeleton of the heart across the aortic leaflet of the mitral valve, and supports the leaflets of the aortic valve in the area of aortomitral continuity. The lateral quadrant of the outflow tract is again muscular and consists of the lateral margin of the inner curvature of the heart, delineated externally by the transverse sinus. The left bundle of the cardiac conduction system enters the left ventricular outflow tract

posterior to the membranous septum and immediately beneath the commissure between the right and noncoronary leaflets of the aortic valve. After traveling a short distance down the septum, the left bundle divides into anterior, septal, and posterior divisions.

THE AORTIC VALVE

The aortic valve is a semilunar valve, morphologically similar to the pulmonary valve (Fig. 9). Because of its central location, the aortic valve is

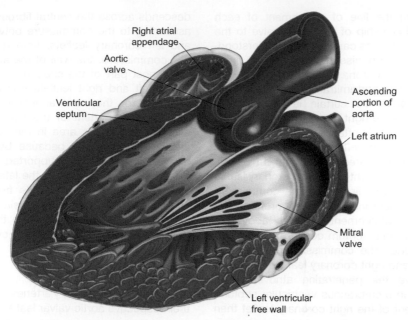

Fig. 8. Characteristic structures of the left ventricle in relation to the left atrium and the aortic valve.

related to each of the cardiac chambers and valves. The aortic valve consists primarily of 3 semilunar leaflets. The attachments of the leaflets extend across the ventriculoarterial junction in a curvilinear fashion. Each leaflet has attachments to the aorta and within the left ventricle. Behind each leaflet, the aortic wall bulges outward to form the sinuses of Valsalva. The leaflets meet centrally along a line of coaptation, at the center of which is a thickened nodule, called the nodule of Arantius. During systole, the leaflets are pushed upward and away from the center of the aortic lumen, whereas, during diastole, they fall passively into the center of the aorta. With normal valvular morphology, all 3 leaflets meet along lines of coaptation and support the column of blood within the aorta to prevent regurgitation into the ventricle. Two of the 3 aortic sinuses of Valsalva give rise to coronary arteries, from which arise their designations as the right, left, and noncoronary sinuses.

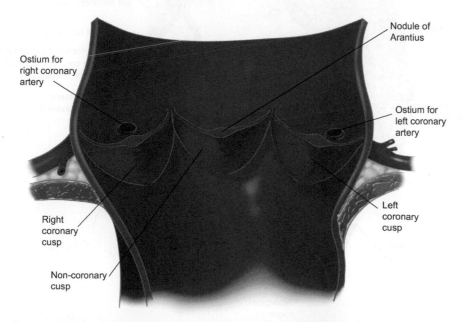

Fig. 9. The ventriculoaortic junction shows the semilunar attachments of the leaflets of the aortic valve.

By following the line of attachment of each leaflet, the relationship of the aortic valve to the surrounding structures can be clearly understood. Posteriorly, the commissure between the non-coronary and left coronary leaflets is positioned along the area of aortomitral valvular continuity. The fibrous subaortic curtain is beneath this commissure. To the right of this commissure, the noncoronary leaflet is attached above the posterior diverticulum of the left ventricular outflow tract. Here the valve is related to the right atrial wall. Because the attachment of the noncoronary leaflet ascends from its nadir toward the commissure between the noncoronary and right coronary leaflets, the line of attachment is directly above the portion of the atrial septum containing the atrioventricular node. The commissure between the noncoronary and right coronary leaflets is located directly above the penetrating atrioventricular bundle and the membranous ventricular septum. The attachment of the right coronary leaflet then descends across the central fibrous body before ascending to the commissure between the right and left coronary leaflets. Immediately beneath this commissure, the wall of the aorta forms the uppermost part of the subaortic outflow. As the facing left and right leaflets descend from this commissure, they are attached to the outlet muscular component of the left ventricle. Only a small part of this area in the normal heart is a true outlet septum because both pulmonary and aortic valves are supported on their own sleeves of myocardium. As the lateral part of the left coronary leaflet descends from the facing commissure to the base of the sinus, it becomes the only part of the aortic valve that is not intimately related to another cardiac chamber.

CORONARY ARTERIES

The right and left coronary arteries originate behind their respective aortic valvar leaflets (**Fig. 10**). The

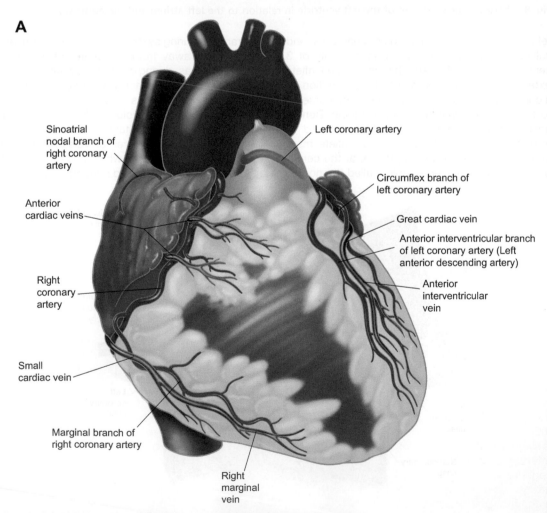

A

Sinoatrial nodal branch of right coronary artery

Left coronary artery

Circumflex branch of left coronary artery

Anterior cardiac veins

Great cardiac vein

Anterior interventricular branch of left coronary artery (Left anterior descending artery)

Right coronary artery

Anterior interventricular vein

Small cardiac vein

Marginal branch of right coronary artery

Right marginal vein

Fig. 10. (*A*) Anterior view of the coronary arterial and venous anatomy.

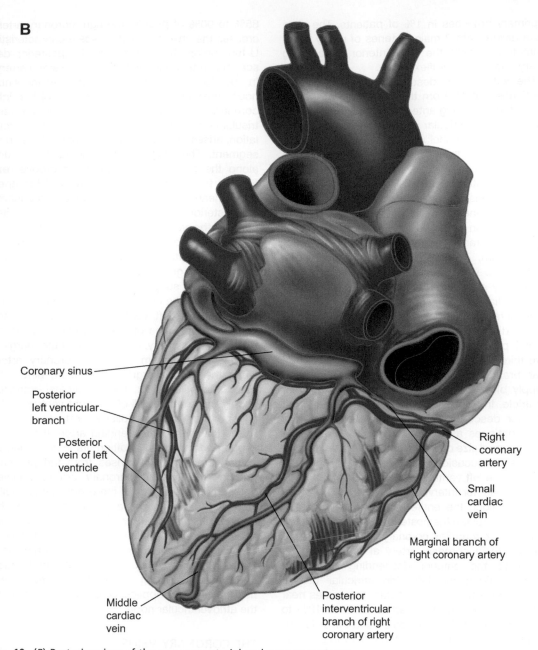

B

Coronary sinus

Posterior
left ventricular
branch

Posterior
vein of left
ventricle

Right
coronary
artery

Small
cardiac
vein

Marginal branch of
right coronary artery

Middle
cardiac
vein

Posterior
interventricular
branch of right
coronary artery

Fig. 10. (*B*) Posterior view of the coronary arterial and venous anatomy.

orifices are typically located in the upper third of the sinuses of Valsalva, although marked variations can be present. Because of the oblique plane of the aortic valve, the orifice of the left coronary artery is superior and posterior to that of the right coronary artery. The coronary arterial tree is divided into 3 segments because the left anterior descending artery and the circumflex artery arise from a common stem, with the right coronary artery as the third segment. The dominance of the coronary circulation refers to the artery from which the posterior descending artery originates. Right dominance is present in 85% to 90% of normal individuals.

The main stem of the left coronary artery courses from the left sinus of Valsalva anteriorly, inferiorly, and to the left between the pulmonary trunk and the left atrial appendage. Typically, it is 10 to 20 mm in length, but can extend to a length of 40 mm. The left main stem can be absent, with separate orifices in the sinus of Valsalva for its

2 primary branches in 1% of patients. The main stem divides into 2 major arteries of nearly equal diameter, namely the left anterior descending artery and the circumflex artery.

The left anterior descending coronary artery continues directly from the bifurcation of the left main stem, coursing anteriorly and inferiorly in the anterior interventricular groove to the apex of the heart. Its branches include the diagonals, the septal perforators, and the right ventricular branches. The diagonals, which may be 2 to 6 in number, course along the anterolateral wall of the left ventricle and supply this portion of the myocardium. The first diagonal is generally the largest and may arise from the bifurcation of the left main stem. The septal perforators branch perpendicularly into the ventricular septum. Typically there are 3 to 5 septal perforators, with the first being the largest and commonly originating just beyond the takeoff of the first diagonal. This perpendicular orientation is a useful marker for identification of the left anterior descending artery on coronary angiograms. The septal perforators supply blood to the anterior two-thirds of the ventricular septum. Right ventricular branches, which are not always present, supply blood to the anterior surface of the right ventricle. In approximately 4% of hearts, the left anterior descending artery bifurcates proximally and continues as 2 parallel vessels of approximately equal size down the anterior interventricular groove. On occasion, the artery wraps around the apex of the left ventricle to feed the distal portion of the posterior interventricular groove. Rarely, it extends along the entire length of the posterior groove to replace the posterior descending artery.

The left circumflex coronary artery arises from the left main coronary artery at roughly a right angle to the anterior descending branch. It courses along the left atrioventricular groove and, in 85% to 95% of patients, terminates near the obtuse margin of the left ventricle. In 10% to 15% of patients, it continues around the atrioventricular groove to the crux of the heart to give rise to the posterior descending artery (left dominance). The primary branches of the left circumflex coronary artery are the obtuse marginals. They supply blood to the lateral aspect of the left ventricular myocardium, including the posteromedial papillary muscle. Additional branches supply blood to the left atrium and, in 40% to 50% of hearts, the sinus node. When the circumflex coronary artery supplies the posterior descending artery, it also supplies the atrioventricular node.

The right coronary artery courses from the aorta anteriorly and laterally before descending in the right atrioventricular groove and curving posteriorly at the acute margin of the right ventricle. In 85% to 90% of people, the right coronary artery crosses the crux, where it makes a characteristic U-turn before bifurcating into the posterior descending artery and the right posterolateral artery. In 50% to 60% of hearts, the artery to the sinus node arises from the proximal portion of the right coronary artery. The blood supply to the atrioventricular node, in patients with right dominant circulation, arises from the midportion of the U-shaped segment. The posterior descending artery runs along the posterior interventricular groove, extending for a variable distance toward the apex of the heart. It gives off perpendicular branches, the posterior septal perforators, that course anteriorly in the ventricular septum. Typically, these perforators supply the posterior one-third of the ventricular septal myocardium. The right posterolateral artery gives rise to a variable number of branches that supply the posterior surface of the left ventricle. The circulation of the posteroinferior portion of the left ventricle is variable. It may consist of branches of the right coronary artery, the circumflex artery, or both. The acute marginal arteries branch from the right coronary artery along the acute margin of the heart, before its bifurcation at the crux. These marginal branches supply the anterior wall of the right ventricle. The right coronary artery supplies important collaterals to the left anterior descending artery through its septal perforators. In addition, its infundibular, or conus, branch, which arises from the proximal portion of the right coronary artery, courses anteriorly over the base of the ventricular infundibulum and may serve as a collateral to the anterior descending artery. The Kugel artery is an anastomotic vessel between the proximal right coronary artery and the circumflex coronary artery that can also provide a branch that runs through the base of the atrial septum to the crux of the heart, where it supplies collateral circulation to the atrioventricular node.

THE CORONARY VEINS

A complex network of veins drains the coronary circulation (see **Fig. 10**). Extensive collateralization among these veins and the coronary arteries, and the paucity of valves within coronary veins, enables the use of retrograde coronary sinus cardioplegia for intraoperative myocardial protection. The venous circulation can be divided into 3 systems: the coronary sinus and its tributaries, the anterior right ventricular veins, and the thebesian veins.

The coronary sinus predominantly drains the left ventricle and receives approximately 85% of the coronary venous blood. It lies within the posterior atrioventricular groove and empties into the right atrium at the lateral border of the triangle of Koch. The orifice of the coronary sinus is guarded by the crescent-shaped thebesian valve. The named tributaries of the coronary sinus include the anterior interventricular vein, which courses parallel to the left anterior descending artery. Adjacent to the bifurcation of the left main stem, the anterior interventricular vein courses leftward in the atrioventricular groove, where it is referred to as the great cardiac vein. It receives blood from the marginal and posterior left ventricular branches before becoming the coronary sinus at the origin of the oblique vein (of Marshall) at the posterior margin of the left atrium. The posterior interventricular vein, or middle cardiac vein, arises at the apex, courses parallel to the posterior descending coronary artery, and extends proximally to the crux. At this point, this vein drains either directly into the right atrium or into the coronary sinus just before its orifice. The small cardiac vein runs posteriorly through the right atrioventricular groove.

The anterior right ventricular veins travel across the right ventricular surface to the right atrioventricular groove, where they either enter directly into the right atrium or coalesce to form the small cardiac vein. This vein travels down the right atrioventricular groove, around the acute margin, and enters into the right atrium directly or joins the coronary sinus just proximal to its orifice. The thebesian veins are small venous tributaries that drain directly into the cardiac chambers. They exist primarily in the right atrium and right ventricle.

A detailed knowledge of the anatomy of the heart and pericardium is of great importance for thoracic surgeons in their clinical practice, and this is most apparent when performing procedures such as mediastinoscopy, resection of mediastinal masses, and pneumonectomy. As cardiac and thoracic surgery continues to get more specialized and the procedures become less invasive, it is essential to have a thorough working knowledge of cardiothoracic anatomy.

FURTHER READINGS

Braunwald E. Essential atlas of heart diseases. Philadelphia: Current Medicine; 1997.

Buxton B, Frazier OH, Westaby S. Ischemic heart disease: surgical management. London: Mosby; 1999.

Cohn LH, Edmunds LH. Cardiac surgery in the adult. 2nd edition. New York: McGraw-Hill; 2003.

Runge MS, Ohman EM. Netter's cardiology. Teterboro (NJ): MediMedia; 2004.

Anatomy of the Thoracic Aorta and of Its Branches

François Dagenais, MD, FRCS(C)

KEYWORDS

- Thoracic aorta • Double arch • Subclavian artery
- Kommerell diverticulum

The thoracic aorta arises from the left ventricle at the level of the third sternocostal joint. The thoracic aorta then courses upward, slightly to the right up to the level of the second sternocostal joint where it arches obliquely to the left and posteriorly to reach the inferior border of the fourth thoracic vertebra. Subsequently, the thoracic aorta descends in the posterior mediastinum to the left side of the T5-T12 vertebrae at which level it penetrates the aortic hiatus in the diaphragm.

Considering its 3 different orientations, the thoracic aorta has been subdivided into 3 sections: the ascending aorta, the aortic arch, and the descending aorta. Each segment has several branches and specific relationships with surrounding structures.

For surgeons performing chest operation, thorough knowledge of the anatomy of the thoracic aorta and of its branches are essential not only to ensure the preservation of adequate organ vascular supply during reconstructive surgery of the esophagus or trachea but also to avoid injury to important thoracic vascular structures. This knowledge of the anatomy of the aorta and of its branches is of paramount importance especially for surgeons performing operations for mediastinal disorders or tumors to avoid catastrophic complications.

ASCENDING AORTA

The ascending aorta (**Fig. 1**) lies within the fibrous pericardium, and at that level, the main pulmonary trunk and ascending aorta are enclosed in a tube of serosal pericardium. The pulmonary infundibulum and the right auricle lie anterior to the lower portion of the aorta, with only the pericardium and thymus remnants separating it from the sternum superiorly. The dome of the left atrium and the right pulmonary artery are contiguous to the posterior aspect of the ascending aorta and form the posterior wall of the transverse sinus, while the superior vena cava and main pulmonary artery are located, respectively, on the right and left sides of the ascending aorta. Beneath the serous pericardium between the aorta and the main pulmonary artery lie lymphatic vessels and the cardiac plexus.

The ascending aorta length averages 5 to 7 cm, and it has a width of 2.5 to 3.0 cm. The ascending aorta is divided into 2 sections: the aortic root and the tubular ascending aorta. The aortic root begins at the aortic annulus and ends at the sinotubular junction where the tubular portion of the ascending aorta begins. The aortic root comprises the aortic annulus, the aortic valve, the sinuses of Valsalva, and the origins of the coronary arteries. The complex interrelationship of these structures is essential to ensure a competent aortic valve.[1,2] Three aortic sinuses are named according to their relationship with the coronary arteries: the right, the left, and the noncoronary sinuses. In 1% of the population, the aortic valve is bicuspid, in which case only 2 aortic sinuses are present. The diameter of the sinotubular junction in normal individuals is approximately 85% of the diameter of the aortic annulus. The tubular portion of the ascending aorta extends up to the level of the

Department of Cardiac Surgery, Institut Universitaire de Cardiologie et de Pneumologie de Laval, Laval Hospital, 2725, Chemin Sainte-Foy, Quebec G1V 4G5, Canada
E-mail address: francois.dagenais@chg.ulaval.ca

Thorac Surg Clin 21 (2011) 219–227
doi:10.1016/j.thorsurg.2010.12.004
1547-4127/11/$ – see front matter © 2011 Elsevier Inc. All rights reserved.

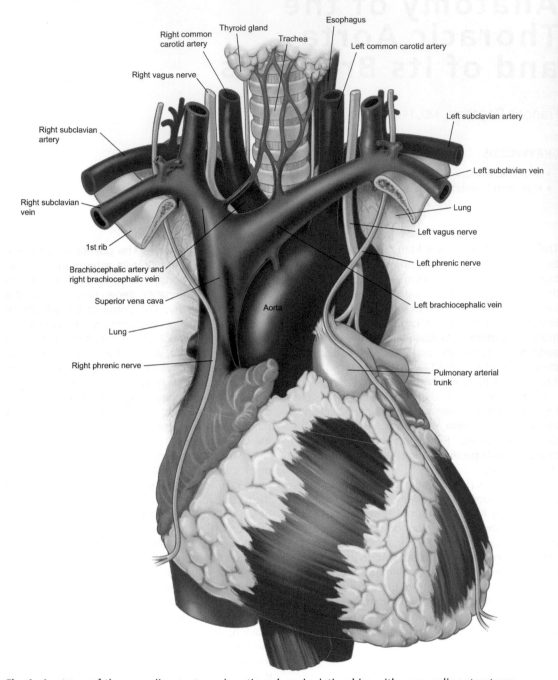

Fig. 1. Anatomy of the ascending aorta and aortic arch and relationships with surrounding structures.

inferior border of the first left sternocostal junction. No branch arises from the tubular portion of the ascending aorta.

AORTIC ARCH AND ITS BRANCHES

Once it exits the pericardium, the ascending aorta gives rise to the aortic arch, which lies beneath the lower half of the manubrium. Initially, the aortic arch ascends diagonally to the left over the anterior portion of the trachea and subsequently descends to the left of the fourth thoracic vertebral body to continue on as the descending component of the thoracic aorta. Variations in arch anatomy are frequent and its relationships with the surrounding structures are complex.[3] Anterior to and to the left of the arch lies the left mediastinal pleura, and deep to the pleura, the arch is crossed anteroposteriorly by the left phrenic nerve, left lower cervical cardiac branch of the vagus nerve, left cervical cardiac branch of the sympathetic trunk, and left vagus nerve (see **Fig. 1**). At the level of the ligamentum arteriosum, the left recurrent nerve branch from the vagus nerve hooks around the left border of the ligamentum and ascends obliquely to the superior portion of the distal arch. Posterior to the arch from right to left lie the trachea and deep cardiac plexus, the left recurrent nerve, the esophagus, the thoracic duct, and the vertebral column. At this level, the arch has a concave shape owing to the imprints of the trachea and the esophagus (**Fig. 2**). The pulmonary artery bifurcation is apposed to the lower

portion of the arch. The ligamentum arteriosum, remnant of the ductus arteriosus, links the lower portion of the arch either to the main or left pulmonary artery. Viewed from the left side, the concavity of the arch represents the upper limit through which structures gain access to the left lung hilum (**Fig. 3**).

The superior convex portion of the arch gives rise anterior-posteriorly to 3 arterial trunks: the brachiocephalic (innominate) artery, the left common carotid artery, and the left subclavian artery. The origins of these arteries are crossed anteriorly by the brachiocephalic vein (see **Fig. 1**). The innominate artery, approximately 5 cm in length, arises behind the midportion of the manubrium and

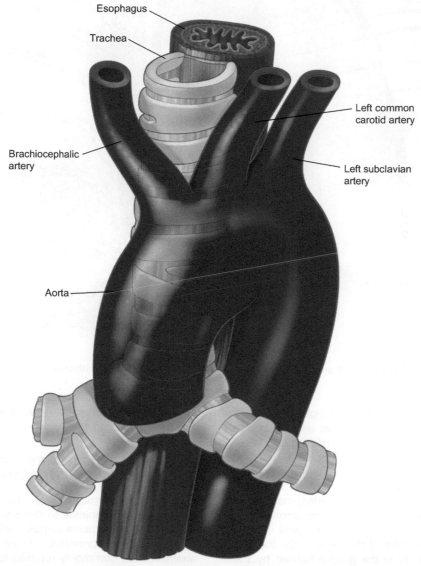

Esophagus

Trachea

Left common
carotid artery

Brachiocephalic
artery

Left subclavian
artery

Aorta

Fig. 2. Aortic arch and great vessels and their relationship with the trachea and esophagus.

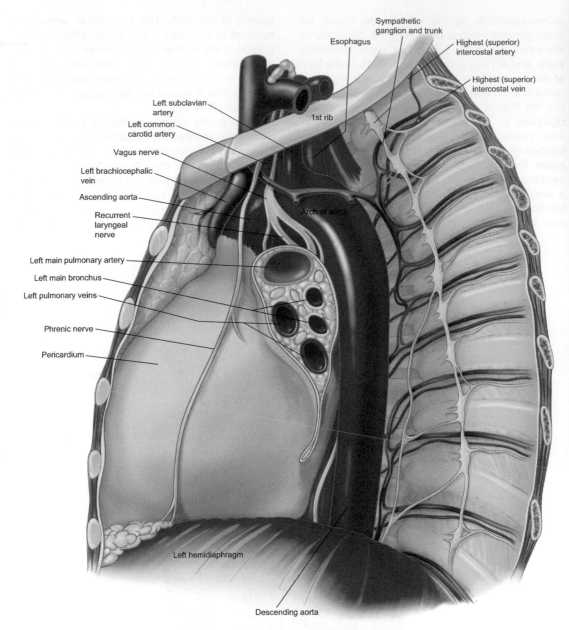

Left subclavian artery

Left common carotid artery

Vagus nerve

Left brachiocephalic vein

Ascending aorta

Recurrent laryngeal nerve

Left main pulmonary artery

Left main bronchus

Left pulmonary veins

Phrenic nerve

Pericardium

Left hemidiaphragm

Descending aorta

Esophagus

Sympathetic ganglion and trunk

Highest (superior) intercostal artery

Highest (superior) intercostal vein

1st rib

Arch of aorta

Fig. 3. View of the aortic arch and descending thoracic aorta from the left hemithorax.

then ascends obliquely to the right in front of the trachea to divide into the right subclavian artery and right common carotid artery at the level of the right sternoclavicular joint. The brachiocephalic artery usually has only terminal branches, although, occasionally, the thyroid ima artery, a thymic artery, or a bronchial artery may originate from this artery. The left common carotid and left subclavian arteries follow a semispiral course to reach the left side of the neck, while the vagus nerve descends in the groove formed by these 2 arteries. Posterior to the left tracheal border lie

the left recurrent laryngeal nerve, the esophagus, and the thoracic duct.

CONGENITAL ABNORMALITIES OF THE AORTIC ARCH AND OF ITS BRANCHES

Congenital abnormalities of the aortic arch system are of pertinence to the thoracic surgeon because they can cause symptomatic tracheal or esophageal compression. These congenital anomalies are commonly referred to as vascular rings.

The double arch model proposed by Edwards[4] is based on the presence of paired fourth aortic arches during embryonic development. Abnormal regression or persistence of portions of this ring results in variations in the anatomy of the thoracic aorta.[5]

Left Aortic Arch

The most common configuration of the thoracic aorta is a combination of left aortic arch, left descending aorta, and left ligamentum arteriosum. The usual pattern of the arch branches

(innominate, left carotid, and left subclavian) is found in 65% to 83% of the population.[6] Anomalies of aortic arch branches include a single common branch and more commonly 2 branches with the left common carotid arising from the innominate artery (bovine arch, 7%–27% of the general population). The right subclavian and right carotid arteries may originate directly from the arch in which case the right subclavian artery arises from the distal end of the arch and courses posterior to the esophagus (**Fig. 4**). Such an aberrant right subclavian artery is considered to be the

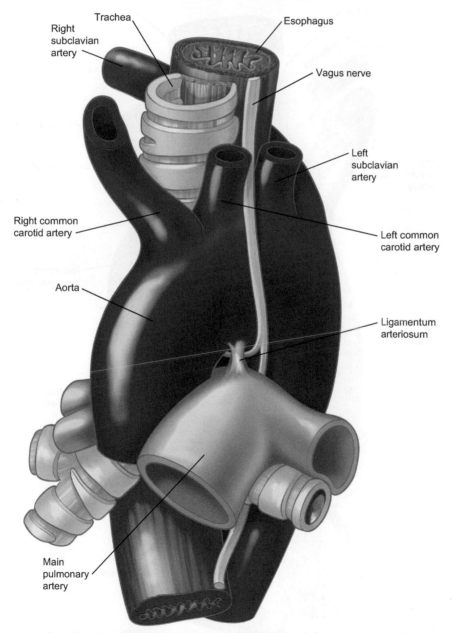

Fig. 4. Aberrant right subclavian artery originating from the proximal descending aorta (Kommerell diverticulum) and coursing posterior to the esophagus.

commonest malformation of the aortic arch and is seen in 1 of every 200 individuals.[7] The origin of such an aberrant right subclavian artery is often dilated and is termed diverticulum of Kommerell. This anomaly is generally asymptomatic in adulthood, although esophageal compression (dysphagia lusoria) may occur when the aberrant artery has become aneurysmal. Numerous abnormalities of the vertebral arteries have been described mainly on the left side with the left vertebral artery originating between the left carotid

and left subclavian arteries in 1%–5% of cadaver dissections.[8]

Right Aortic Arch

A right-sided arch occurs in 0.1% of the normal population.[9] This anomaly is divided into 5 subgroups, and type 3 is most commonly seen in the adult population, which consists of a right arch with an aberrant left subclavian artery (**Fig. 5**). In this variety, the right-sided aortic arch gives off

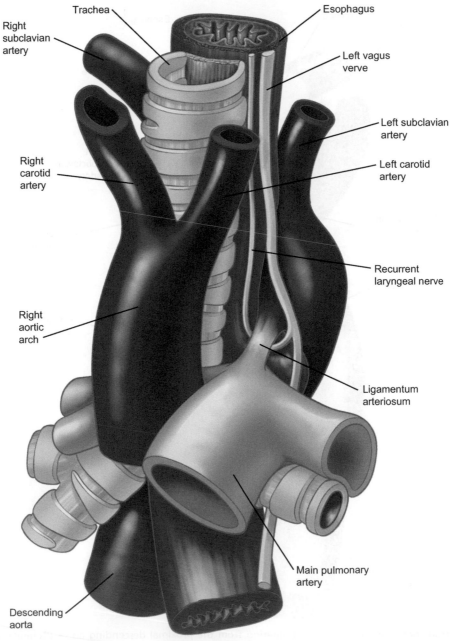

Fig. 5. Type 3 right aortic arch.

successively the left common carotid, the right carotid, the right subclavian, and finally an aberrant left subclavian artery, which arises from a Kommerell diverticulum in the descending aorta and courses posterior to the trachea and esophagus. The descending aorta is more commonly right sided. If there is a patent left ligamentum arteriosum between the posteriorly located left subclavian artery and the left pulmonary artery, a vascular ring is formed and symptoms are related to the tightness of the ring (see **Fig. 4**).

Double Aortic Arch

A double aortic arch (**Fig. 6**) is present in 0.3% of postmortem examinations and is the most

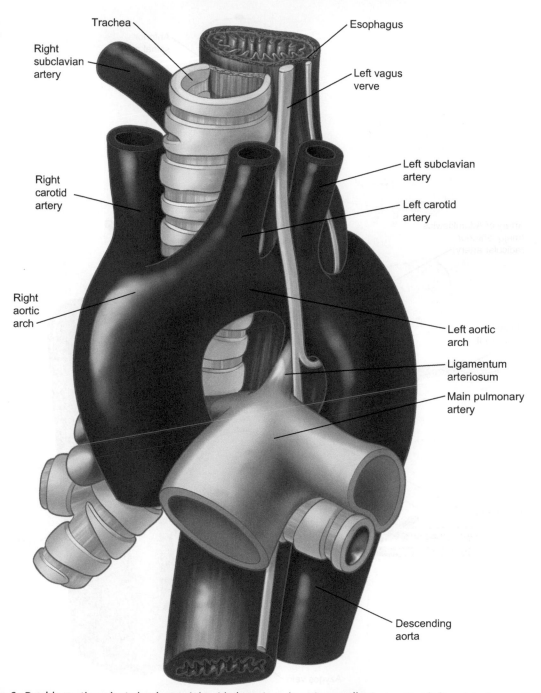

Fig. 6. Double aortic arch. A dominant right-sided aortic arch with a smaller but patent left arch is shown. Each arch gives rise to its respective carotid and subclavian arteries.

common cause of complete vascular ring.[10] In most cases, both arches are patent, the right arch generally being higher and larger than the left. The arch crosses over posteriorly to the trachea and esophagus to join the descending aorta, which is usually left sided. Each arch gives rise to its respective carotid and subclavian arteries. Symptoms of dysphagia or tracheal obstruction are usually present during childhood, although in 25% of cases, the diagnosis is only made during adulthood.

DESCENDING THORACIC AORTA

The descending thoracic aorta, in continuity with the arch, begins at the lower border of the 4th

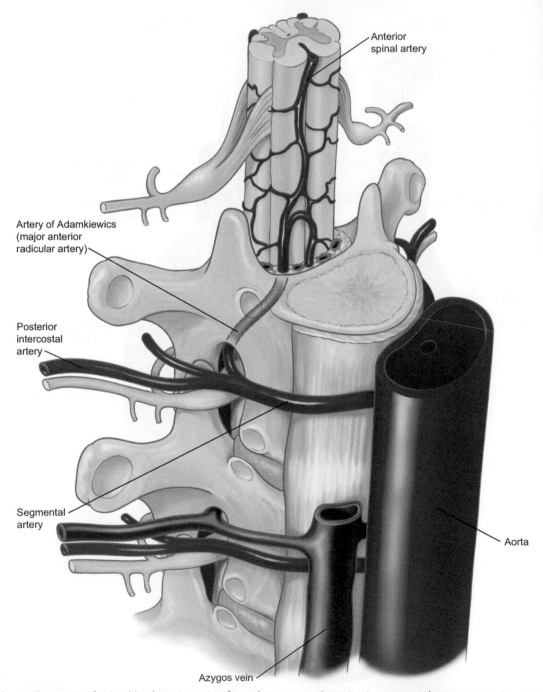

Fig. 7. The artery of Adamkiewicz originating from the posterior branch of a segmental artery. Note the characteristic hairpin turn of the artery before it becomes the anterior spinal artery.

thoracic vertebra and penetrates the diaphragm anterior to the 12th thoracic vertebra. At its origin, the descending thoracic aorta is located on the left side of the spine, but at the level of the 7th thoracic vertebra, it becomes slightly to the right and anterior to the vertebral bodies. In front of the descending aorta, from cephalad to caudal, lie successively the left pulmonary hilum (pulmonary artery, left main bronchus, and inferior pulmonary vein), the pericardium covering the left atrium, the esophagus, and the diaphragm. Located posteriorly are the vertebral column and the hemiazygos vein, whereas the azygos vein and thoracic duct lie on its right lateral side. Further lateral are the right pleura and lung while the left lateral side is bordered by the left pleura and lung. The esophagus, which spirals around the aorta, is located in a right anterolateral position superiorly, becomes anterior in the lower chest, and goes to a left anterolateral position at the level of the diaphragm.

The descending thoracic aorta gives branches to the pericardium, bronchi, chest wall, and esophagus. Bronchial arteries vary in number, size, and origin. The usually single right bronchial artery does not originate directly from the thoracic aorta, but rather from the third posterior intercostal artery or from the upper left bronchial artery. Two left bronchial arteries usually arise from the descending aorta, the upper near the fifth thoracic vertebra and the lower below the level of the left main bronchus. A few small pericardial and mediastinal branches also originate from the descending aorta and irrigate the posterior aspect of the pericardium and areolar tissues and lymph nodes of the posterior mediastinum. From the lower thoracic descending aorta arise branches, which are distributed posterior to the superior surface of the diaphragm.

Of the 11 posterior intercostal arteries, 9 originate from the descending aorta, whereas the first and second arteries arise from the superior intercostal artery, which is a branch of the costocervical trunk of the subclavian artery. The right posterior intercostal arteries course directly over the vertebral bodies and are covered by the right pleura. The left posterior intercostal arteries course posterior to the hemiazygos and splanchnic nerves and then divide into the anterior and posterior rami.

The T8-L1 intercostal arteries are important for the vascular supply of the lower portion of the spinal cord. The great artery of Adamkiewicz (**Fig. 7**) usually arises from a left intercostal artery in the T8-L1 region. This artery then divides into a small upper anterior spinal artery and a larger lower spinal artery, which supplies the anterior portion of the lower spinal cord. The concept of a single Adamkiewicz artery is debated because the artery can be identified in only 86% of individuals by angiography,[11]

and it may be double in certain patients. However, clinical data support the importance of the contribution of the T8-L1 intercostal arteries to the vascular supply of the lower spinal cord.

Subcostal arteries are the last paired branches of the descending thoracic aorta. Each one runs laterally to the 12th thoracic vertebral body and enters the abdomen posterior to the arcuate ligament. Each artery courses posterior to the colon on each side, perforates the aponeurosis of the transverses abdominis muscle, and anastomoses with the superior epigastric artery.

SUMMARY

Knowledge of the relationship between the thoracic aorta and intrathoracic organs is essential to select appropriate incisions and to safely expose diseased structures. In this context, the adult thoracic surgeon must be familiar with the normal anatomy of the thoracic aorta as well as with the main congenital anomalies of the aortic arch.

REFERENCES

1. Anderson RH. Anatomy: clinical anatomy of the aortic root. Heart 2000;84:670–3.
2. Hopkins RA. Aortic valve leaflet sparing and salvage surgery: evolution of technique for aortic root reconstruction. Eur J Cardiothorac Surg 2003;24:886–97.
3. Das SK, Byrom R. Aortic root anomalies of the neck presenting in adults. Review of the literature with three case reports. Eur J Vasc Endovac Surg 2005;30:48–51.
4. Edwards JE. Anomalies of the derivatives of the aortic arch system. Med Clin North Am 1948;32:925.
5. VanDyke CW, White RD. Congenital abnormalities of the thoracic aorta presenting in the adult. J Thorac Imaging 1994;9:230–45.
6. Gray's anatomy. Philadelphia: Elsevier Churchill Livingstone; 2005. p. 1023.
7. Klinkhamer AC. Esophagography in anomalies of the aortic arch syndrome. Baltimore (MD): Williams and Wilkins Co; 1969. p. 16–30.
8. Vorster W, Du Plooy PT, Meiring JH. Abnormal origin of internal thoracic and vertebral arteries. Clin Anat 1998;11:33–7.
9. Hastreiter AR, D'Cruz IA, Chantez T. Right-sided aorta. Part 1. Occurrence of right aortic arch in various types of congenital heart disease. Br Heart J 1966;28:722–5.
10. Glew D, Hartnell GG. The right aortic arch revisited. Clin Radiol 1991;43:305–7.
11. Kieffer E, Fukui S, Chira J, et al. Spinal cord arteriography: a safe adjunct before descending thoracic or thoracoabdominal aortic aneurysmectomy. J Vasc Surg 2002;35:262–8.

Anatomy of the Thoracic Duct

Hamid Hematti, MD[a], Reza J. Mehran, MD[b],*

KEYWORDS

- Thoracic duct • Lymphatic capillaries • Vertebra
- Cisterna chyli

ANATOMY OF THE THORACIC DUCT

The thoracic duct is a major anatomic structure of the upper part of abdomen, chest, and the lower part of the neck. A precise knowledge of the anatomy of the duct is essential in the safe performance of any surgical procedures involving these areas.

Lymphatic capillaries are joined from the most remote parts of the interstitium by tissue channels, many of which are only a few tens of microns long. These channels form collecting systems that are many centimeters long and drain lymph from the initial lymphatic capillary into the venous system.[1] Lymphatic capillaries consist of single layers of flat endothelial cells, which are slightly larger and thinner than blood capillary cells. Basement membrane is absent or vestigial, which allows large molecules to permeate the wall easily.[2] Because of their greater permeability lymphatic capillaries are more effective than blood capillaries in removing protein-rich fluid from the intercellular spaces.

When the collected fluid enters the lymphatic vessels, it is called lymph. The lymphatic vessels also serve to transport proteins and lipids that are too large to cross the fenestrations of the absorptive capillaries of the small intestine. Before returning to the blood, lymph passes through lymph nodes, where it is exposed to the cells of the immune system.[3] The lymphatic vessels merge to create the thoracic duct, which drains the lymph toward the venous system at the base of the left part of the neck at a volume estimated to be 1.38 mL/kg of the body weight per hour.[4] Because of this large volume of lymph, understanding the complex anatomy of the thoracic duct is key to preventing traumatic chylothorax.

EMBRYOLOGY

The lymphatic system begins forming in the human embryo during the sixth week of development when the embryo is about 10 mm in length. These first lymphatics are blunt buds, which are located near the internal jugular veins at the root of the neck.[5] At the end of the embryonic period, there are 6 primary lymph sacs: 2 jugular lymph sacs, 2 iliac lymph sacs, 1 retroperitoneal lymph sac, and 1 cisterna chyli (**Fig. 1**). Lymphatic vessels develop in a manner similar to blood vessels and join the lymph sacs.[6] Linkage of the jugular lymph sacs with the cisterna chyli, the abdominal origin of the thoracic duct, is initially in the form of a bilateral system of lymphatic trunks, connected with one another across the midline by numerous collateral anastomoses. Of these trunks, the inferior portion of the right trunk and the superior portion of the left trunk, together with a diagonal anastomosing channel at the level of T4-T6 segments, forms the definitive thoracic duct[7]; the rest of the ducts regress with time. Except for the superior part of the cisterna chyli, the lymph sacs are transformed into groups of lymph nodes during the early fetal period.[6] The uppermost lymph node to form is generally called the Virchow node and is located at or near the jugulosubclavian venous junction.[8]

---

[a] Department of Thoracic and Cardiovascular Surgery, The University of Texas MD Anderson Cancer Center, 1515 Holcombe Boulevard, Houston, TX 77030, USA

[b] Department of Thoracic and Cardiovascular Surgery, Unit 445, The University of Texas MD Anderson Cancer Center, 1515 Holcombe Boulevard, Houston, TX 77030, USA

* Corresponding author.

E-mail address: rjmehran@mdanderson.org

Thorac Surg Clin 21 (2011) 229–238
doi:10.1016/j.thorsurg.2011.01.002

thoracic.theclinics.com

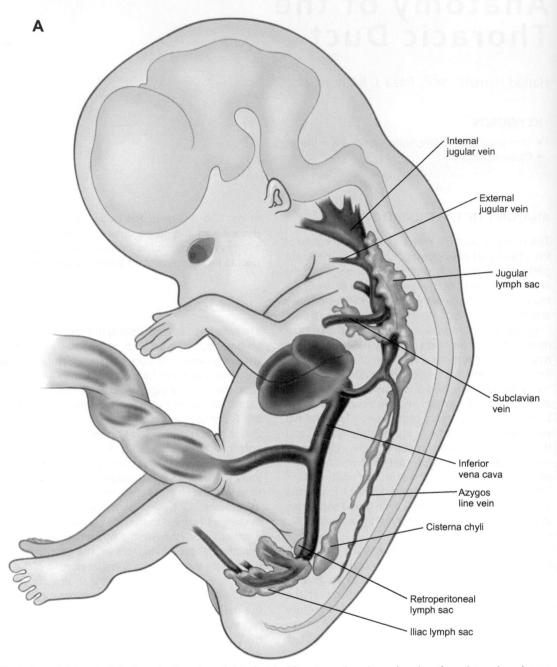

Fig. 1. Development of the lymphatic system. (*A*) Left side of an 8-week embryo showing the primary lymph sacs. (*B*) Ventral view of the lymphatic system at and after 9 weeks' gestation, showing the paired thoracic ducts and the regression of the left duct. (*Adapted from* Moore KL, Persaud TVN. The developing human. 7th edition. Philadelphia: WB Saunders; 2003; with permission.)

CISTERNA CHYLI AND ABDOMINAL LYMPH TRUNKS

The 4 main abdominal lymph trunks converge to form an elongated arrangement of channels referred to as the abdominal confluence of lymph trunks or the cisterna chyli (see **Fig. 1**). To further complicate matters, this group of channels may have a simple ductlike structure or may be duplicated, triplicated, or plexiform.[9] A fusiform area of dilatation in the lymphatic channels, which extends 5 to 7 cm in the caudocephalad direction,

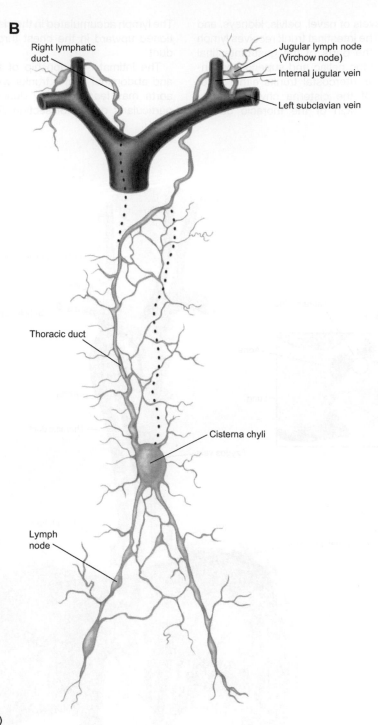

B

Right lymphatic duct

Jugular lymph node (Virchow node)

Internal jugular vein

Left subclavian vein

Thoracic duct

Cisterna chyli

Lymph node

Fig. 1. (*continued*)

has been reported in 53% of lymphangiographic studies,[10] 50% of autopsies,[11] and 15% of abdominal magnetic resonance imaging studies.[12]

The cisterna chyli is generally found along the vertebral column at the L2 level, but it may also be found anywhere between T10 and L3, generally to the right of the aorta.[4] The medial edge of the right crus of the diaphragm lies anterior to the abdominal confluence of lymph trunks. The confluence receives the right and left lumbar trunks and the intestinal lymph trunks.[9] The right and left lumbar trunks deliver lymph from the abdominal wall below the levels of navel, pelvis, kidneys, and adrenal glands. The intestinal trunk receives lymph and chyle from the parts of the gastrointestinal tract supplied by the celiac and superior mesenteric arteries. The intercostal trunks either enter the upper part of the cisterna chyli or empty directly into the origin of the thoracic duct.[13]

The lymph accumulated in the cisterna chyli is suctioned upward in the chest through the thoracic duct.

The intimate relationship of the cisterna chyli and abdominal lymph trunks with the abdominal aorta may lead to injury during aortic surgery, particularly during dissection performed around

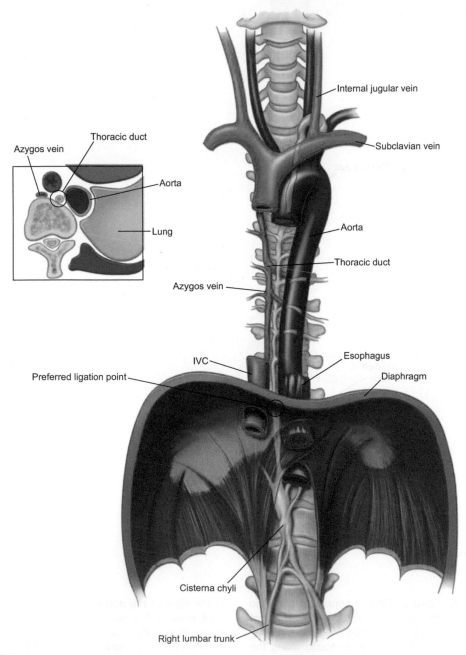

Thoracic duct

Azygos vein

Aorta

Lung

Internal jugular vein

Subclavian vein

Aorta

Thoracic duct

Azygos vein

IVC

Esophagus

Diaphragm

Preferred ligation point

Cisterna chyli

Right lumbar trunk

Fig. 2. Surgical anatomy of thoracic duct showing the preferred point of thoracic duct mass ligation in the surgical treatment of chylothorax. IVC, inferior vena cava.

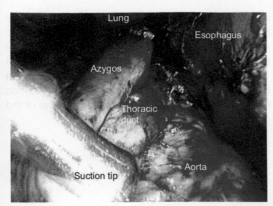

Fig. 3. Location of the thoracic duct in midthoracic cavity after division of the azygos vein during a minimally invasive esophagectomy (the esophagus has been mobilized interiorly in this figure).

the aorta above the level of the celiac axis. The large caliber of the trunks coupled with the volume of lymph flowing through them can lead to problematic chylous (lymphatic) ascites.[9]

THORACIC DUCT

The thoracic duct is the largest lymphatic channel in the body, measuring 38 to 45 cm in length and 2 to 5 mm in diameter. It extends from L2 to the base of the neck (**Fig. 2**). This duct collects lymph from the entire body except from the right sides of the head and neck, right upper hemithorax, and the right upper extremity that are mainly drained by the right lymphatic trunk.[13]

The thoracic duct contains a well-developed basement membrane and has 3 layers within its wall: intima, media, and adventitia. The media consists of smooth muscle fibers supported by connective tissue containing elastic fibers, which contract periodically to aid the lymph flow. The thoracic duct and all lymphatic channels, except the smallest ones, have valves. These valves are more numerous and closer together than the valves of veins. The valves are so close that a distended lymphatic vessel may appear beaded because of dilated sections between the valves.[2]

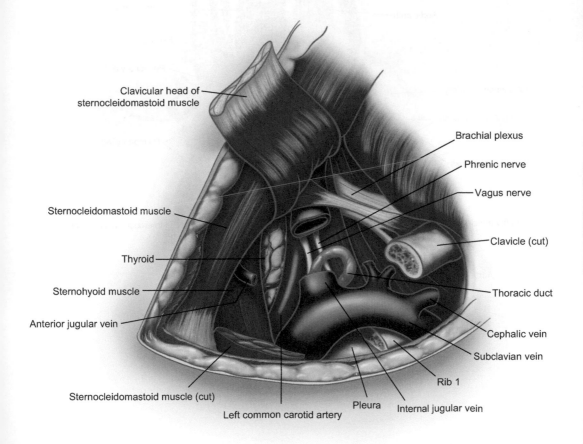

Fig. 4. Termination of the thoracic duct. Note the thoracic duct curving anteriorly to drain into the junction between the internal jugular and left subclavian veins.

The origin of the thoracic duct starts at the superior pole of the cisterna chyli, traverses the aortic hiatus of the diaphragm (see **Fig. 2**), and then ascends the posterior mediastinum, to the right of the midline, between the descending thoracic aorta on the left and the azygos vein on the right (**Fig. 3**). The vertebral column and the right intercostal arteries lie posterior to the thoracic duct. The diaphragm and esophagus are anterior. A recess of the right pleural cavity may separate the duct and the esophagus.

At the T5 level, the duct gradually inclines to the left, enters the superior mediastinum, and ascends toward the thoracic inlet along the left edge of the

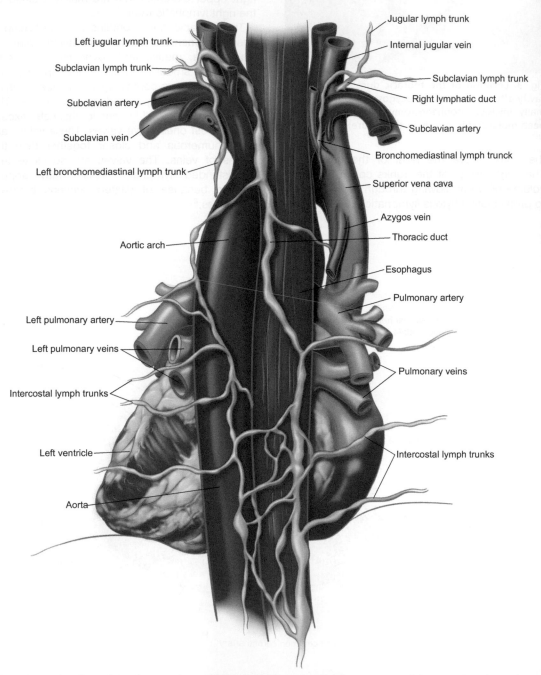

Fig. 5. Posterior view of the thoracic duct and its tributaries Note that the remnant of the right lymphatic duct in the neck forms from the union of 3 lymphatic trunks: right jugular, right subclavian, and right bronchomediastinal trunks.

esophagus. In this part of its course, the duct is first crossed anteriorly by the aortic arch and then runs posterior to the initial segment of the left subclavian artery, in close contact with the left mediastinal pleura. Passing into the neck, the thoracic duct arches laterally at the level of the transverse process of the C7 vertebra. Its arch rises 3 or 4 cm above the clavicle (**Fig. 4**). The duct passes posterior to the left common carotid artery, vagus nerve, and internal jugular vein. Finally, the duct descends anterior to the first part of the left subclavian artery, and after receiving branches from the left sides of the head and neck and from the left upper limb, it most commonly ends by opening into the junction of the left subclavian and internal jugular veins. The duct may also open into either of the great veins, near the junction, or it may divide into several smaller vessels, each terminating individually in the venous system.

The thoracic duct is 0.5 cm in diameter at its abdominal origin. It diminishes in caliber at the midthoracic level but grows to 0.5 cm again before its termination into the jugular vein.[9] The thoracic duct is dilated in several clinical conditions, such as cirrhosis with portal hypertension and right-sided heart failure.[14–17]

Although the diameters of the common bile duct and the pancreas increase during aging, the diameter of the thoracic duct does not seem to do so.[18]

Several tributaries join the thoracic duct at various places along its length (**Fig. 5**). Bilateral descending thoracic lymph trunks from intercostal lymph nodes of the lower 6 or 7 intercostal spaces on both sides traverse the aortic hiatus and join the lateral aspects of the thoracic duct in the abdomen immediately after its origin. Bilateral ascending lumbar lymph trunks from the upper lateral aortic nodes ascend and pierce their corresponding diaphragmatic crura and then join the thoracic duct at various levels within the thorax.

The upper intercostal trunks drain the intercostal nodes in the upper 5 or 6 left intercostal spaces. The left subclavian trunk usually joins the thoracic duct but may open independently into the left internal jugular vein. The left bronchomediastinal trunk occasionally joins the thoracic duct as well but usually has an independent venous opening.[9]

Some thoracic duct tributaries may directly drain lymph from an organ without crossing any lymph node along their course (anodal route). This anodal route has been observed for the diaphragm, the esophagus, and the lower lobes of the lungs.[19] Direct lymphatic drainage of the

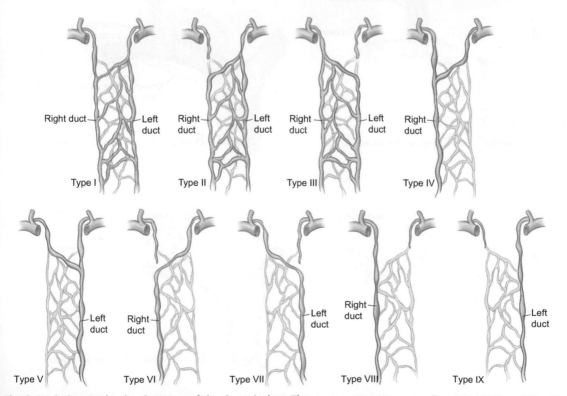

Fig. 6. Variations in the development of the thoracic duct. The most common types are Type VI at 63% and Type II at 27%. (*Adapted from* Davis HK. A statistical study of the thoracic duct in man. Am J Anat 1915;17:211–44; with permission.)

esophagus into the thoracic duct has also been identified macroscopically in as many as 19.8% to 22.7% of cadavers.[20–22] The drainage pattern may play an important role in the prognosis of cancers involving these organs and may help explain the poor prognosis of esophageal cancer and the possibility of distant metastases in non–small cell lung cancer, even when there is no lymph node involvement.

RIGHT LYMPHATIC TRUNK

The right lymphatic trunk in the neck typically forms from the union of 3 lymphatic trunks: right jugular, right subclavian, and right bronchomediastinal trunks (see **Fig. 5**). The right bronchomediastinal trunk is regarded as the vestigial portion of the cranial segment of the embryologic right thoracic duct. It receives lymphatic drainage from the right lung, lower part of the left lung, and right side of the diaphragm; most of the drainage from the heart; and some drainage from the right lobe of the liver.[13] The right lymphatic trunk has a variable anatomy, including a doubling of the duct and left-sided, right-sided, or bilateral termination.

ANATOMIC VARIATIONS OF THE THORACIC DUCT

Although a thorough understanding of the anatomy of the thoracic duct is essential when performing procedures within the thoracic cavity to prevent the complication chylothorax, the "textbook" anatomy of the thoracic duct is found in only 50% of individuals. In the other 50% of cases, the thoracic duct anatomy may vary considerably.

Variations in Origin

As described earlier, the right and left lumbar lymphatic trunks arise from several roots and converge to form the thoracic duct. The junction lies between L2 and T12 vertebrae. A cisterna chyli is present when the junction is low at the level of the lumbar vertebral bodies. When the junction is higher than the 12th vertebra, there may be dilation of both lumbar trunks, which perhaps represents the unfused lateral primordia of the cisterna, or there may be no trace of a cisterna. A cisterna is present in about 50% of adults examined.[7]

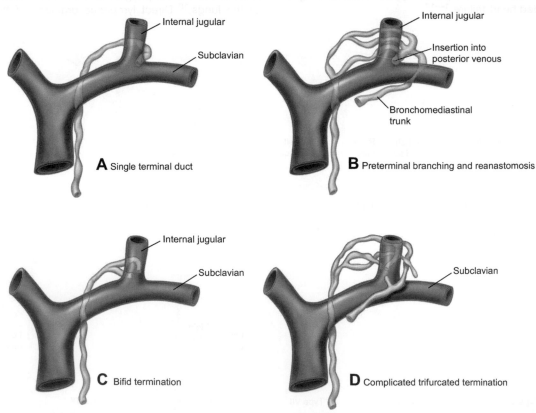

Fig. 7. Variations in termination of the thoracic duct. (*A*) Typical termination of the thoracic duct (single terminal duct). (*B*) Preterminal branching and reanastomosis of the thoracic duct. (*C*) Bifid termination. (*D*) Complicated trifurcated termination.

Variations in Anatomy

In 1915, Davis[11] first proposed 9 types of anatomic variations of the thoracic duct (**Fig. 6**). These variations depend on which portion of the embryonic thoracic duct atrophies and disappears and which portion continues to develop. In the anatomic study by Davis, which was based on the dissection of 22 cadavers, it was found that the most frequent anatomic variation of the thoracic duct is a doubling of the lower part of the duct caused by the persistence of both right and left trunks. Even when a single trunk has formed, the contralateral trunk is usually not completely absent and is connected by numerous cross-anastomoses to the main trunk. In addition, the thoracic duct may itself break into a plexus of lymphatic vessels, which reunite to form a single channel higher in the thorax.[7] In a larger series, the incidence of doubling was reported between 39% and 47%.[4] Complete bilateral thoracic ducts with coexistent persistent left superior vena cava[23] and termination of the thoracic duct in the azygos system are some examples of rare variations reported in the literature.[4]

Variations in Termination

The thoracic duct empties into the left great veins of the neck in 92% to 95% of cases, on the right side of the neck in 2% to 3% of cases, and bilaterally in 1.0% to 1.5% of cases.[24] The duct can have a superior extension above the clavicle, as much as 5 cm in 8.3% of cases, that predisposes it to surgical damage.[25] The thoracic duct terminates in the venous system as a single vessel in 68% to 87.5% of cases, as 2 ducts in 8.33% to 25% of cases, and as 3 terminal branches in 4.2% to 7% of cases (**Fig. 7**).[13,25] In about 20% of cases, thoracic ducts show branching and reanastomosing patterns before termination.[25]

The final termination patterns of the thoracic duct vary greatly. According to different observers, the final drainage site of the terminal branches of the thoracic duct is the junction of the left subclavian and internal jugular veins in about 7.5% to 64.3% of cases, the internal jugular vein in 4.8% to 85% of cases, the external jugular vein in 7.1% to 28% of cases, and the subclavian vein in 3.6% to 57.1% of cases.[9,13,25–28]

REFERENCES

1. Casley-Smith JR. The importance of the lymphatic system. Angiology 1985;36:201–2.
2. Fortin D, Incult RI, Malthaner RA. The thoracic duct and chylothorax. In: Patterson GA, Cooper JD, Pearson FG, editors. Pearson's thoracic & esophageal surgery. 3rd edition. Philadelphia: Elsevier Health Sciences; 2008. p. 1108–20.
3. Ross MH, Pawlina W. Cardiovascular system. In: Histology: a text and atlas with correlated cell and molecular biology. 5th edition. Baltimore (MD): Lippincott; 2006. p. 364–86.
4. Miller JI Jr. Anatomy of the thoracic duct and chylothorax. In: Shields TW, LoCicero J, Ponn RB, et al, editors. General thoracic surgery. 6th edition. Philadelphia: Lippincott; 2005. p. 879–88.
5. Sabin FR. The method of growth of the lymphatic system. Science 1916;14:145–58.
6. Moore KL, Persaud TV. The cardiovascular system. In: The developing human: clinically oriented embryology. 7th edition. Philadelphia: WB Saunders; 2003. p. 329–80.
7. Skandalakis JE, Gray SW. Lymphatic system. In: Skandalakis JE, Gray SW, Ricketts RR, editors. Embryology for surgeons. 2nd edition. Baltimore (MD): Williams & Wilkins; 1994. p. 877–97.
8. Mizutani M, Nawata S, Hirai I, et al. Anatomy and histology of Virchow's node. Anat Sci Int 2005;80: 193–8.
9. Shah P. Heart and mediastinum. In: Standring S, editor. Gray's anatomy. 39th edition. Edinburgh (UK): Elsevier Churchill Livingstone; 2005. p. 977–94.
10. Rosenberger A, Abrams HL. Radiology of the thoracic duct. Am J Roentgenol Radium Ther Nucl Med 1971;111:807–20.
11. Davis HK. A statistical study of the thoracic duct in man. Am J Anat 1915;17:211–44.
12. Pinto PS, Sirlin CB, Andrade-Barreto OA, et al. Cisterna chyli at routine abdominal MR imaging: a normal anatomic structure in the retrocrural space. Radiographics 2004;24:809–17.
13. Skandalakis JE, Skandalakis LJ, Skandalakis PN. Anatomy of the lymphatics. Surg Oncol Clin N Am 2007;16:1–16.
14. Dumont AE, Mulholland JH. Alterations in thoracic duct lymph flow in hepatic cirrhosis: significance in portal hypertension. Ann Surg 1962;156:668–75.
15. Zironi G, Cavalli G, Casali A, et al. Sonographic assessment of the distal end of the thoracic duct in healthy volunteers and in patients with portal hypertension. Am J Roentgenol 1995;165: 863–6.
16. Parasher VK, Meroni E, Malesci A, et al. Observation of thoracic duct morphology in portal hypertension by endoscopic ultrasound. Gastrointest Endosc 1998;48:588–92.
17. Takahashi H, Kuboyama S, Abe H, et al. Clinical feasibility of noncontrast-enhanced magnetic resonance lymphography of the thoracic duct. Chest 2003;124:2136–42.
18. Parasher VS, Bhutani MS. Can age alter the thoracic duct diameter? An endosonographic study. Am J Gastroenterol 2001;96:S28–9.

19. Riquet M, Barthes FL, Souilamas R, et al. Thoracic duct tributaries from intrathoracic organs. Ann Thorac Surg 2002;73:892–8.

20. Kuge K, Murakami G, Mizobuchi S, et al. Submucosal territory of the direct lymphatic drainage system to the thoracic duct in the human esophagus. J Thorac Cardiovasc Surg 2003;125:1343–9.

21. Murakami G, Sato I, Shimada K, et al. Direct lymphatic drainage from the esophagus into the thoracic duct. Surg Radiol Anat 1994;16:399–407.

22. Deslauriers J, Mehran R. Management of post operative complications after pulmonary surgery. In: Handbook of perioperative care in general thoracic surgery. Philadelphia: Elsevier Health Sciences; 2008. p. 303–99.

23. Chen HY, Shoumura S, Emura S. Bilateral thoracic ducts with coexistent persistent left superior vena cava. Clin Anat 2006;19:350–3.

24. Gottwald F, Finke C, Zenk J. Thoracic duct cysts: a rare differential diagnosis. Otolaryngol Head Neck Surg 2005;132:330–3.

25. Langford RJ, Daudia AT, Malins TJ. A morphological study of the thoracic duct at the jugulo-subclavian junction. J Craniomaxillofac Surg 1999; 27:100–4.

26. Kinnaert P. Anatomical variations of the cervical portion of the thoracic duct in man. J Anat 1973; 115:45–52.

27. Shimada K, Sato I. Morphological and histological analysis of the thoracic duct at the jugulo-subclavian junction in Japanese cadavers. Clin Anat 1997;10:163–72.

28. Jdanov DA. [Anatomie du canal thoracique et des prencipaux collecteurs lymphatiques du tronc chez l'homme]. Acta Anat (Basel) 1959;37:20–47 [in French].

Nerves of the Mediastinum

Jingyi Wang, MD[a,b], Ji Li, MD[a], Guojin Liu, MD[b],
Jean Deslauriers, MD, FRCS(C)[c],*

KEYWORDS
- Nerve anatomy • Mediastinum • Thoracic neoplasm

The most important nerves of the mediastinum are the phrenic and vagus nerves, the thoracic spinal nerves, the sympathetic trunks and ganglia, and the autonomic plexuses. Thorough knowledge of their normal anatomy and of their variants cannot be overestimated because nerve trauma during thoracic surgical procedures can have catastrophic consequences. For instance, recurrent nerve damage is associated with vocal cord dysfunction and higher overall mortality after pulmonary resection.[1,2] Damage to the phrenic nerve results in complete paralysis and eventual atrophy of the corresponding half of the diaphragm. In individuals with 2 lungs, such paralysis is associated with the loss of approximately 75% of respiratory efficiency on the affected side,[3,4] whereas in patients undergoing pneumonectomy, it has recently been shown[5] that the long-term effects of a paralyzed ipsilateral hemidiaphragm are characterized by significant alterations in expiratory lung volumes and exercise tolerance.

Knowledge of mediastinal nerve anatomy is also important because mediastinal or lung tumors can locally infiltrate those nerves either directly or through nodal metastases, making them generally unresectable.

PHRENIC NERVES

The phrenic nerves are formed in the neck at the lateral border of the anterior scalenus muscles, chiefly from the C4 nerve roots but also with contributions from the C3 and C5 nerve roots. From there, they enter the superior mediastinum between the ipsilateral subclavian artery and innominate vein and pass anterior to the pulmonary hilum along the pericardium (**Fig. 1**A, B). Each nerve is accompanied in its course through the thorax by pericardiacophrenic arteries and veins of the internal mammary vessels. Both nerves divide into several terminal branches at the level of the corresponding hemidiaphragm or just above.

Right Phrenic Nerve

In the thorax, the right phrenic nerve passes caudally over the cupula of the pleura and descends posterolaterally along the right side of the right brachiocephalic vein and external surface of the superior vena cava. It then passes in front of the right hilum (see **Fig. 1**A) over the right side of the pericardium and descends along the upper part of the inferior vena cava to the diaphragm, where it branches.

Left Phrenic Nerve

The left phrenic nerve is slightly longer than its right counterpart and it descends between the left common carotid and subclavian arteries, crossing in front of the left vagus nerve.[6] It then passes lateral to the aortic arch and descends in front of the left

a Heilongjian Provincial Hospital, Haerbin, 250036 People's Republic of China
b First Teaching Hospital, Changchun, Jilin Province, 130021, People's Republic of China
c Institut Universitaire de Cardiologie et de Pneumologie de Québec, Laval University, 2725 Chemin Sainte-Foy, Quebec City, Quebec G1V 4G5, Canada
* Corresponding author.
E-mail address: jean.deslauriers@chg.ulaval.ca

Thorac Surg Clin 21 (2011) 239–249
doi:10.1016/j.thorsurg.2011.01.006

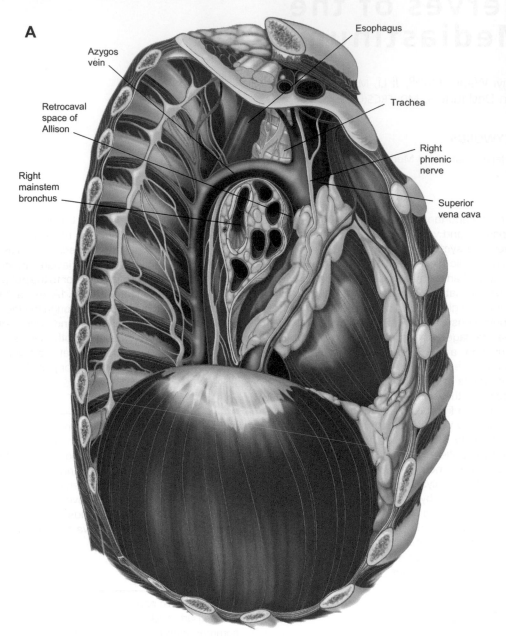

Fig. 1. (*A*) Diagram showing right phrenic nerve and hilum of right lung. Note that the right phrenic nerve descends along the external surface of the superior vena cava then passes in front of the right hilum.

hilum (see **Fig. 1**B) to the diaphragm, where it branches. At the level of the aortic arch, the left phrenic nerve, which has a near vertical course along the pericardium, has a more oblique direction (**Fig. 2**).

Accessory Phrenic Nerves

The accessory phrenic nerves are minute branches that arise from or are a continuation of the subclavian nerves (nerve to subclavious

B

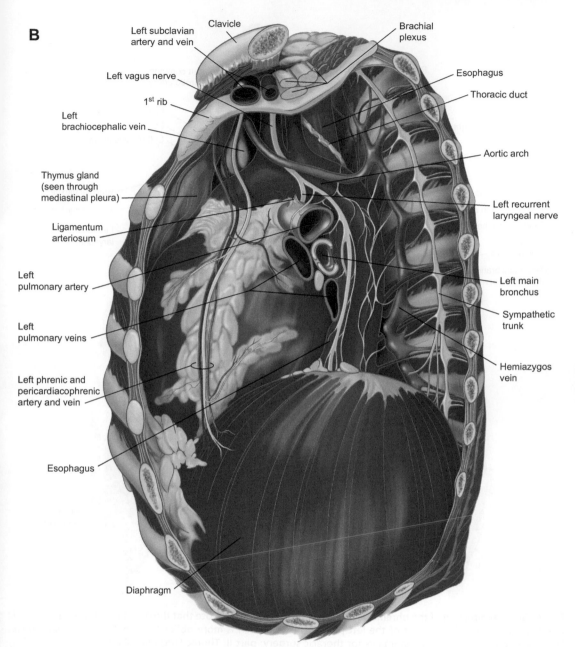

Clavicle

Left subclavian
artery and vein

Brachial
plexus

Left vagus nerve

Esophagus

Thoracic duct

1st rib

Left
brachiocephalic vein

Aortic arch

Thymus gland
(seen through
mediastinal pleura)

Left recurrent
laryngeal nerve

Ligamentum
arteriosum

Left
pulmonary artery

Left main
bronchus

Sympathetic
trunk

Left
pulmonary veins

Hemiazygos
vein

Left phrenic and
pericardiacophrenic
artery and vein

Esophagus

Diaphragm

Fig. 1. (*B*) Left phrenic nerve and hilum of left lung. Note that the left phrenic nerve passes lateral to the aortic arch and descends in front of the left hilum.

muscles). They join the main phrenic nerve trunks at the base of the neck or high into the thorax, and are present in approximately 20% to 30% of normal individuals. These accessory nerves usually descend in front of the subclavian vein as opposed to the main phrenic nerves that pass behind it. If the phrenic nerves are surgically damaged in the neck, the accessory phrenic nerves, when present, may still provide motor function to the diaphragm.

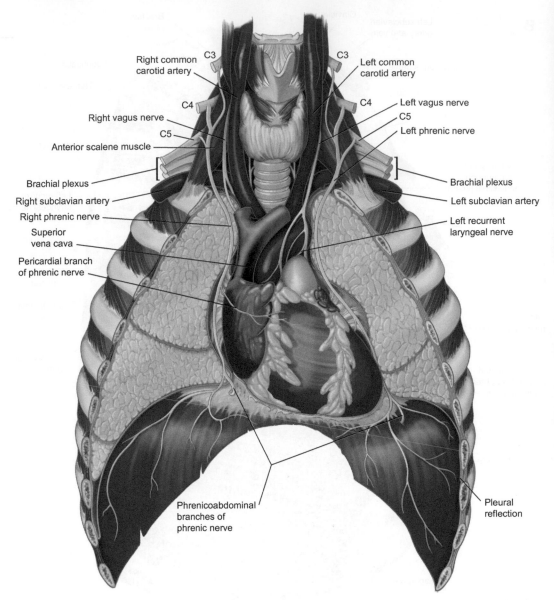

Fig. 2. General direction of the phrenic nerves along the pericardium. Note that the direction of the right phrenic nerve is more vertical than that of the left phrenic nerve, which is more oblique. (*From* Smith SE, Darling GE. Surface anatomy and surface landmarks for thoracic surgery: part II. Thorac Surg Clin 2011;21(2).

Diaphragmatic Branching of the Phrenic Nerves

The phrenic nerves divide at the level of the diaphragm or just above it into several terminal branches, which were described by Merendino in 1954.[7,8] Because this branching arrangement is constant and predictable, surgical incisions in the diaphragm that are protective of the nerves can safely be performed.[9]

In most individuals, there are 3 muscular branches that arise from each phrenic nerve (**Fig. 3**), and these are named the sternal or anterior branch (directed anteromedially toward the sternum), the anterolateral branch, and the posterolateral branch. The crural or posterior

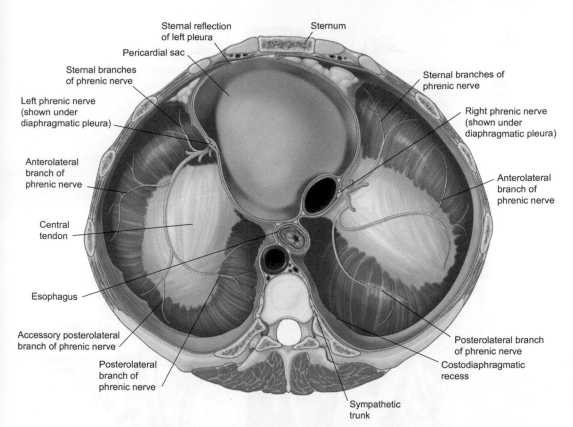

Fig. 3. Main branches of the phrenic nerves at the level of the diaphragm. Incisions made in a circumferential manner in the periphery of the diaphragm do not involve the section of any significant branches of the phrenic nerves.

branch, which extends dorsomedially to the region of the diaphragmatic crura, arises from the posterolateral branch. All of these branches are usually located deep in the muscle rather than lying exposed on the undersurface of the diaphragm.

VAGUS NERVE

The vagus nerves leave the skull through the jugular foramen anterior to the jugular vein. They then proceed caudally through the neck within the carotid sheath behind the internal carotid artery and internal jugular vein. Each nerve enters the superior mediastinum behind its respective sternoclavicular joint and branchiocephalic vein.

Right Vagus Nerve and Recurrent Laryngeal Nerve

At the base of the neck, the right vagus nerve crosses the origin of the right subclavian artery behind the sternoclavicular joint, where it gives off the right recurrent laryngeal nerve (inferior laryngeal nerve), which loops around and under the artery (**Fig. 4**A, B). The right recurrent laryngeal nerve reaches the tracheoesophageal groove behind the common carotid artery, where it can be injured during cervicomediastinal dissections performed for tumors located at the thoracic inlet.

In the thorax, the right vagus nerve runs posteriorly through the superior mediastinum on the right side of the trachea. It then passes posteromedial to the right brachiocephalic vein, superior vena cava, and pulmonary hilum, where it divides into posterior pulmonary branches that unite with rami from the thoracic sympathetic ganglia to form the right pulmonary plexuses. It then continues onto the esophagus, where it forms the esophageal plexus (**Fig. 5**) with the left vagus nerve. At the lower end of the esophagus, these plexuses collect into an anterior and a posterior vagal trunk, which descend into the abdomen alongside the esophagus.

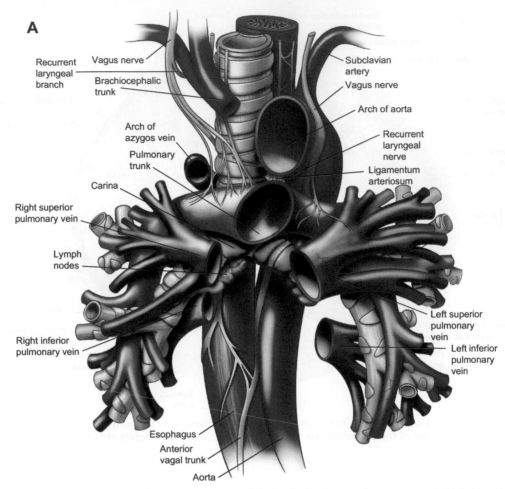

A

Recurrent laryngeal branch

Vagus nerve

Brachiocephalic trunk

Arch of azygos vein

Pulmonary trunk

Carina

Right superior pulmonary vein

Lymph nodes

Right inferior pulmonary vein

Subclavian artery

Vagus nerve

Arch of aorta

Recurrent laryngeal nerve

Ligamentum arteriosum

Left superior pulmonary vein

Left inferior pulmonary vein

Esophagus

Anterior vagal trunk

Aorta

Fig. 4. (*A*) Course of the vagus and recurrent nerves and their relationships to the great vessels. ([*A*] *From* Minnich DJ, Mathisen DJ. Anatomy of the trachea, carina, and bronchi. Thorac Surg Clin 2007;17(4):571–85; with permission.)

Left Vagus Nerve and Recurrent Laryngeal Nerve

The left vagus nerve enters the mediastinum between the left common carotid and left subclavian arteries. When it reaches the aortic arch, it curves posteriorly, crossing to the left side of the arch. The left recurrent laryngeal nerve originates from the vagus nerve as it curves medially at the inferior border of the arch (see **Fig. 4**A, C). It hooks below the arch, lateral to the ligamentum arteriosum, and ascends to the larynx in the groove between the trachea and the esophagus. At the left hilum, the vagus nerve contributes to the pulmonary plexuses and then enters the esophageal plexuses, where it joins with rami from the right vagus nerve.

THORACIC SPINAL NERVES

After emerging from the intervertebral foramen below the corresponding vertebra, each thoracic spinal nerve divides into a dorsal and ventral ramus (**Fig. 6**), a ramus communicant through which it connects with the sympathetic trunk and a smaller ramus meningeus that returns to the spinal canal. The dorsal ramus runs posteriorly and supplies the muscles, bones, joints, and skin of the back. Each dorsal ramus divides into a medial cutaneous branch and a lateral muscular branch.

The ventral ramus of the first 11 thoracic spinal nerves is called the intercostal nerve. Each nerve enters the intercostal space behind the endothoracic fascia and parietal pleura and in front of the superior costotransverse ligament. The ventral

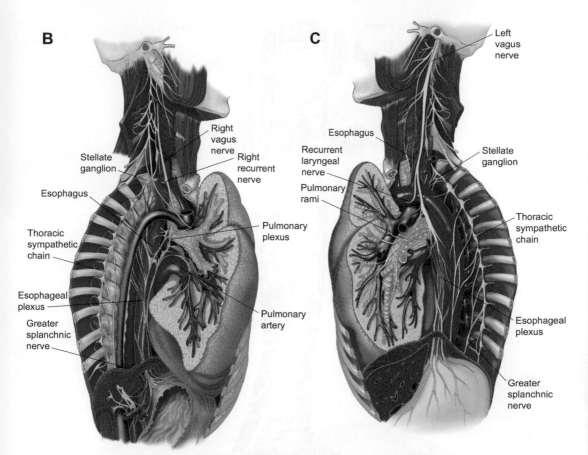

Fig. 4. (*B*) Anatomy of the right vagus nerve. (*C*) Anatomy of the left vagus nerve.

ramus of the 12th spinal nerve is called the sub-costal nerve.

SYMPATHETIC TRUNKS AND GANGLIA

The thoracic sympathetic trunks are located ventral to the heads of the ribs and behind the endothoracic fascia and parietal pleura. They enter the abdomen by piercing the diaphragm or behind the medial arcuate ligaments and they join the lumbar sympathetic trunks.

The first thoracic sympathetic ganglia is usually fused with the inferior cervical ganglia to form the cervicothoracic ganglion located anterior to the transverse process of C7 just superior to the neck of the first rib. The length of this ganglia is approximately 8 mm and although it is named the stellate ganglia, its shape can be variable. The vertebral artery and vein are located in front of the

cervicothoracic ganglia. There are 11 other small thoracic ganglia, which generally lie at the level of the corresponding intervertebral disc. They are interconnected through segments of the main trunks and each connects with the corresponding ventral ramus of the spinal nerve through 2 or more rami communicantes.

SPLANCHNIC NERVES

The splanchnic nerves arise form the thoracic sympathetic trunks (**Fig. 7**). The greater splanchnic nerves are formed by rami from the fifth to the ninth thoracic ganglia and they descend obliquely on the vertebral bodies to form unique trunks at approximately the level of the 10th thoracic vertebra. These trunks perforate the ipsilateral crus of the diaphragm to end in the celiac ganglia.

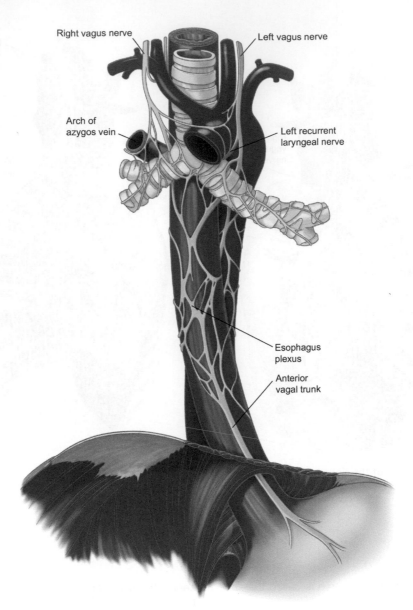

Fig. 5. The esophageal plexuses.

The lesser splanchnic nerves are formed by inferior rami originating from the 10th to the 12th thoracic sympathetic ganglia. They descend lateral and behind the greater splanchnic nerves. After piercing the diaphragm, they end in the renal plexuses.

MAJOR THORACIC PLEXUSES
Pulmonary Plexuses

The pulmonary plexuses (see **Fig. 7**) are located anterior and posterior to the hilar structures of the lungs and they are interconnected. The anterior plexus is poorly developed and formed by rami from the vagus nerves and cervical sympathetic cardiac nerves, whereas the larger posterior plexus is formed by rami from vagal cardiac branches and from the second to the sixth thoracic sympathetic ganglia. When they exit the pulmonary plexuses, the nerves pass into the pulmonary parenchyma, where they divide into periarterial and peribronchial plexuses.

Cardiac Plexuses

The most widely accepted anatomic description of cardiac innervation consists of 3 major

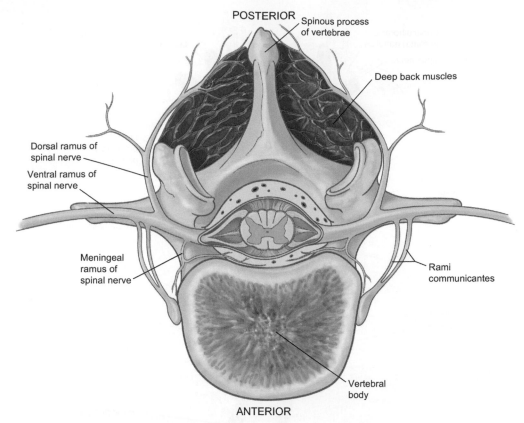

POSTERIOR Spinous process
of vertebrae

Deep back muscles

Dorsal ramus of
spinal nerve

Ventral ramus of
spinal nerve

Meningeal
ramus of
spinal nerve

Rami
communicantes

Vertebral
body

ANTERIOR

Fig. 6. Branching of thoracic spinal nerves.

sympathetic cardiac nerves arising from the superior cervical ganglia, middle cervical ganglia, and stellate ganglia. These sympathetic nerves together with a similar number of parasympathetic cardiac nerves innervate the heart via the cardiac plexuses,[10] which lie mainly under the epicardium. In 1984, this anatomy was reinvestigated by Janes and colleagues[11] because the previous descriptions were inconsistent and differed markedly from those of subhuman primates.

All major sympathetic cardiopulmonary nerves were found to arise from the stellate ganglia and the caudal halves of the cervical sympathetic trunks below the level of the cricoid cartilage. These sympathetic cardiopulmonary nerves usually consist of 3 nerves on the right side and 4 on the left. In contrast to widely accepted reports, no sympathetic cardiopulmonary nerves were found to arise from the superior cervical ganglia or the thoracic sympathetic trunks inferior to the stellate ganglia. Parasympathetic cardiopulmonary nerves were found to arise from the recurrent laryngeal nerves and

the thoracic vagi immediately distal to them. These nerves interconnect with sympathetic cardiopulmonary nerves anterior and posterior to the main pulmonary artery to form the ventral and dorsal cardiopulmonary plexuses. These plexuses contain relatively large nerves as well as smaller interconnections. Emerging from these plexuses to innervate the ventricles are 3 distinct relatively large cardiac nerves: the right and left coronary cardiac nerves and left lateral cardiac nerve. In addition to these 3 major nerves, small cardiac nerves arise from the plexuses and the thoracic vagi.

Esophageal Plexuses

These plexuses are formed by the vagus nerves after they leave the pulmonary plexuses. At the lower end of the esophagus, the plexuses located in front of the esophagus collect into an anterior vagal trunk, whereas those behind the esophagus collect into a posterior vagal trunk.

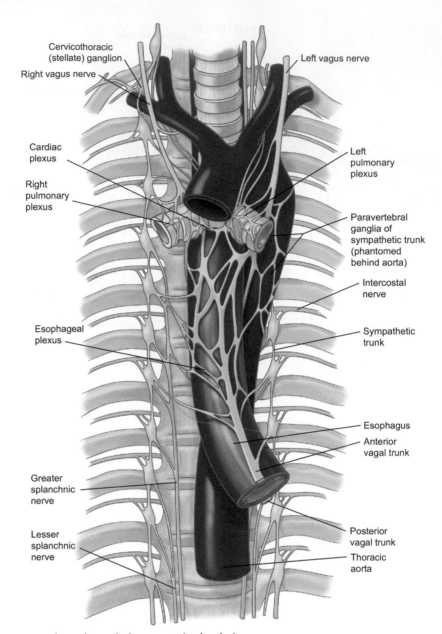

Fig. 7. Pulmonary and esophageal plexuses and splanchnic nerves.

SUMMARY

Knowledge of the anatomy of mediastinal nerves is essential for the evaluation and surgical treatment of most thoracic neoplasms. Familiarity with this anatomy helps the surgeon to better understand thoracic diseases and prevent potentially major intraoperative and postoperative complications.

REFERENCES

1. Filaire M, Mom T, Laurent S, et al. Vocal cord dysfunction after left lung resection for cancer. Eur J Cardiothorac Surg 2001;20:705–11.
2. Myssiorek D. Recurrent laryngeal nerve paralysis: anatomy and etiology. Otolaryngol Clin North Am 2004;37:25–44.

3. Agostini E, Sant'Ambrogia G. The diaphragm. In: Campbell E, Agostini E, Newson DJ, editors. The respiratory muscles, mechanics and neurological control. London: Lloyd-Luke; 1970. p. 145–60.

4. Clague HW, Hall DR. Effect of posture on lung volume: airway closure and gas exchange in hemidiaphragmatic paralysis. Thorax 1979;34: 523–6.

5. Ugalde P, Miro S, Provencher S, et al. Ipsilateral diaphragmatic motion and lung function in long-term pneumonectomy patients. Ann Thorac Surg 2008; 86:1745–52.

6. Fell SC. Surgical anatomy of the diaphragm and the phrenic nerve. Chest Surg Clin N Am 1998;8: 281–94.

7. Merendino KA, Johnson RJ, Skinner HH, et al. The intradiaphragmatic distribution of the phrenic nerve with particular reference to the placement of diaphragmatic incisions and controlled segmental paralysis. Surgery 1956;39:189–98.

8. Merendino KA. The intradiaphragmatic distribution of the phrenic nerve. Surgical significance. Surg Clin North Am 1964;44:1217–26.

9. Schumpelick V, Steinav G, Schluper I, et al. Surgical embryology and anatomy of the diaphragm with surgical applications. Surg Clin North Am 2000;80: 213–39.

10. Hurst JW, editor. The heart, vol. 1. New York: McGraw-Hill; 1982. p. 1018.

11. Janes RD, Brandys JC, Hopkins DA, et al. Anatomy of human extrinsic cardiac nerves and ganglia. Am J Cardiol 1986;57:299–309.

FURTHER READINGS

Cordier G, Delmas AH. Rouvière, Anatomie Humaine, Tome 2: Tronc. 9e édition. Paris: Masson; 1962.

Gardner E, Gary DJ, O'Rahilly R. Anatomy. A regional study of human structure. 3rd edition. Philadelphia: WB Saunders; 1969.

Moore KL, Dalley AF II. Clinically oriented anatomy. 5th edition. Philadelphia: Lippincott Williams & Wilkins; 2006.

Shields TW, Locicero J, Ponn RB, et al. General thoracic surgery. 6th edition. Philadelphia: Lippincott Williams & Wilkins; 2005.

Correlative Anatomy for the Mediastinum

Paula A. Ugalde, MD[a,*], Sergio Tadeu Pereira, MD[a],
Cesar Araujo, MD[b], Klaus Loureiro Irion, MD, PhD, FRCR[c]

KEYWORDS
• Mediastinum • Anatomy • Diagnostic imaging

Diseases of the mediastinum comprise a wide spectrum of benign and malignant entities that share the same anatomic site within the chest. Knowledge of the mediastinum anatomy, pathology of the mediastinal diseases, demographics, clinical presentation, and imaging patterns are indispensable for a correct management, which often requires a multidisciplinary approach. Diagnostic imaging modalities play a major role in the diagnosis of mediastinal diseases and guiding minimally invasive diagnostic procedures, minimizing the risk of imaging guided biopsies. Computed tomography (CT), magnetic resonance imaging (MRI), ultrasonography (US), and positron emission tomography (PET) have completely changed the diagnostic approach, providing exquisite anatomic detail and discrimination between the different components of mediastinal masses as well as their metabolic activity. In addition, CT and US have revolutionized the diagnostic intervention of mediastinal masses, by allowing real-time assessment of needle biopsy or indication of the most appropriate approach for a minimally invasive surgical exploration such as mediastinoscopy or mediastinotomy.

Unsuspected cases of mediastinal diseases are frequently detected by chance, when the patient is submitted to a chest radiograph, by the identification of abnormal mediastinal contour or density. An abnormal mediastinum on chest radiograph must trigger further investigation with CT, MRI, or US (**Fig. 1**). At present, chest radiography can or should be avoided in patients who are suspected of having mediastinal diseases,[1] such as patients with palpable neck nodes, patients with leukemia or lymphoma, patients with symptoms of myasthenia, patients with hemoptysis, or patients with signs of superior vena cava obstruction. In these situations, the lack of sensitivity of the chest radiograph can represent a risk for delaying diagnosis. CT and MRI are indicated as the initial imaging investigation of the mediastinum, obviating chest radiographs.[2,3]

In this article the authors describe the mediastinal anatomy, correlating the findings of plain radiography, CT, and MRI.

OVERVIEW OF THE ANATOMY

The mediastinum is interposed between both pleural cavities and withholds all intrathoracic structures, except the lungs and pleurae. It extends from the inner surface of the sternum to the anterior aspect of the thoracic spine and from the thoracic inlet to the diaphragm.

Over the years, different subdivisions of the mediastinum have been proposed, though none is universally accepted. The approach taken here divides the mediastinum into 3 longitudinal compartments, extending from the level of the thoracic inlet to the level of the diaphragm (**Fig. 2**).

Funding: none.
[a] Department of Thoracic Surgery, Santa Casa de Misericordia Hospital, Praça Cons Almeida Couto, #500, Centro Medico Celso Figueroa, sala 207, Nazaré 40000, Salvador-Ba, Brazil
[b] Department of Radiology, Federal University of Bahia School of Medicine, Rua Augusto Viana s/n - Canela 40110-160, Salvador-Ba, Brazil
[c] Department of Radiology, Liverpool Heart and Chest Hospital, The Royal Liverpool and Broadgreen University Hospital, Liverpool, UK
* Corresponding author.
E-mail address: paugalde@terra.com.br

Thorac Surg Clin 21 (2011) 251–272
doi:10.1016/j.thorsurg.2010.12.008

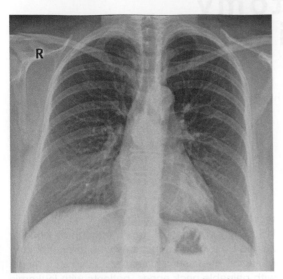

Fig. 1. Chest radiograph with abnormal mediastinum. A subcarinal mass is noted.

The middle mediastinum is a vascular space that contains the heart and pericardium with its other contents, the great vessels, the ascending aorta and aortic arch, its major branches and the brachiocephalic veins, up to the thoracic inlet (**Fig. 3**). Several of the mediastinal nodal stations and portions of the phrenic and vagus nerves are included in the middle mediastinum according to some investigators. The concept of the middle mediastinum as a vascular space excludes the trachea from this compartment, as opposed to other proposed division systems.[1]

The anterior mediastinum is the prevascular space from the thoracic inlet to the point of contact of the heart with the sternum. It includes the thymus, lymph nodes, and internal mammary vessels, and continues in the lower neck containing the thyroid and parathyroid glands.

The posterior mediastinum or "postvascular space" contains the trachea, esophagus, descending aorta, and azygos vein. This space continues into the neck in the plane of the retropharyngeal space and the so-called perivisceral space, which includes the trachea, esophagus, azygos and hemiazygos veins, some nodal stations, and the thoracic duct. It also contains the lower portion of the vagus and sympathetic chains.

It is important to consider that the Fleischner Society glossary of terms states the following[4]:

Nominal anatomic compartments of the mediastinum include the anterior, middle, posterior, and (in some schemes) superior compartments. The anterior compartment is bounded anteriorly by the sternum and posteriorly by the anterior surface of the pericardium, the ascending aorta, and the brachiocephalic vessels. The middle compartment is bounded by the posterior margin of the anterior division and the anterior margin of the posterior division. The posterior compartment is bounded anteriorly by the posterior margins of the pericardium and great vessels and posteriorly by the thoracic vertebral bodies. In the 4-compartment model, the superior compartment is defined as the compartment above the plane between the sternal angle to the T4-5 intervertebral disk or, more simply, above the aortic arch. Exact anatomic boundaries between the compartments do not exist, and there are no barriers (other than the pericardium) to prevent the spread of disease between compartments.

PLAIN CHEST RADIOGRAPHY

Frontal view (F) can be obtained in either anteroposterior projection or posteroanterior projection. Lateral view (L) can be obtained in either right to left or left to right projections. Frontal view (**Fig. 4**) is the basic imaging modality for the assessment of the chest and mediastinum so that it is possible to recognize several structures. Lateral view (**Fig. 5**) is extremely helpful, although not always included in the basic investigation of the chest. Additional projections include oblique views and lordotic projection, and can be helpful, particularly in centers that do not count on the benefit of a CT scanner. Moreover, fluoroscopic examination and opacification of the esophagus can provide valuable additional information.

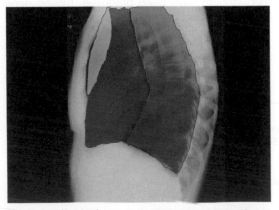

Fig. 2. Mediastinal compartments: anterior or prevascular (*green*), middle or vascular (*red*), and posterior or postvascular (*blue*).

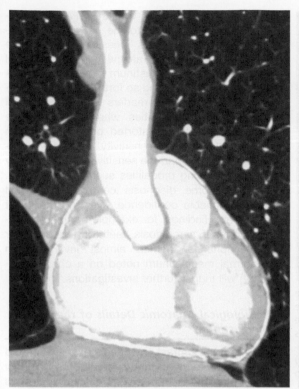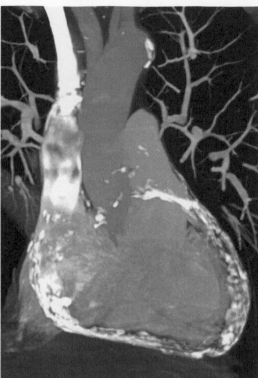

Fig. 3. CT reconstruction of the middle mediastinum: contents of the pericardium and vessels extending to the neck. The pericardium here is calcified, demarcating the lower aspect of the middle mediastinum.

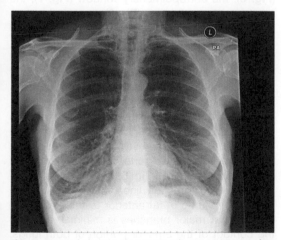

Fig. 4. Frontal chest radiograph. The examination has been acquired with a digital radiograph system (DR) that improves the anatomic detail of the mediastinal landmarks, without compromising the analysis of the lung parenchyma. In this image it is possible to recognize the right paratracheal line, the anterior mediastinal triangle, anterior and posterior mediastinal septum, the azygoesophageal recess, and the aortopulmonary window.

A mediastinal mass will be identified or suspected on chest radiographs by the presence of a distorted mediastinal contour, obliteration of some of the anatomic landmarks such as the paratracheal line or azygoesophageal recess (see **Fig. 1**), or by the presence of abnormal density breaking the usual gradual change in the shade of greys (Dégradé) of the chest radiographs. Mediastinal mass can also be identified by the presence of abnormal calcifications or by displacement of anatomic structures. In many situations, mediastinal diseases course a prolonged asymptomatic phase and, not infrequently, will be detected as an incidental finding on chest radiographs performed for any other reason. As already mentioned, in the presence of clinical signs or symptoms of mediastinal disease the chest radiographs can be obviated in favor of a CT examination as the first imaging investigation modality.

The sensitivity of a chest radiograph reader improves significantly if he or she is aware of the anatomic details that can be depicted by the contrast interface between soft tissue densities of some anatomic structures of the mediastinum

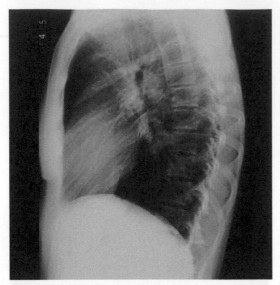

Fig. 5. Normal left lateral chest radiograph. The correct positioning can be assessed by the adequate visualization of the inner and outer margins of the sternal body and by the characteristic appearances of the posterior arch of the ribs. There is a homogeneous gradual change in the shade of grey (dégradé) where the spine gets darker as one looks from top to bottom. It is possible to identify the air in the trachea, in the right and left main bronchi, and in the bronchus intermedius. The posterior wall of the trachea and the posterior wall of the bronchus intermedius are visible as thin lines. Looking carefully, one can identify the arch of the aorta and another arch, distal to the aortic one, which is the arch of the left pulmonary artery, "sitting" on the left main bronchus (dark round structure seen just below the left pulmonary artery). In front of the tracheal carina and of the bronchus intermedius it is possible to identify a denser round structure which is the right pulmonary artery. Note also that the left hemidiaphragm disappears when in contact with the heart as the air-soft tissue contrast interface is then lost. The right hemidiaphragm can be seen from the magnified group of ribs to the anterior chest wall, still visible at the level of the heart.

against the low density of the air within the lungs, airways or esophagus. One should expand observation of the mediastinum beyond the lateral contours traditionally taught in medical schools. The margins of the mediastinum in the chest radiographs are much more complex than the boundaries composed by the superior vena cava and right atrium on the right side and aortic arch, left atrium appendage, and left ventricle on the left side. Digital radiographs provide better density discrimination of the anatomic details of the mediastinum, obviating the necessity of an additional radiographic view with an increased dose previous necessary for the assessment of the mediastinum

in the pre-CT era, which was known as the mediastinum view.[5] Thanks to the new digital radiographic systems it is possible to visualize anatomic details such as the right paratracheal line, the anterior mediastinum triangle, the aortopulmonary window, and so forth, without an additional view.[6] Trained readers can detect small mediastinal abnormalities when one of these anatomic details is distorted or is denser than usual, although the sensitivity of digital radiographs is far beyond the sensitivity and specificity of other imaging modalities such as CT or MRI. Although some diagnosis can be established with reasonable confidence solely on the chest radiograph findings, for example egg-shell calcified nodes in sarcoidosis, teeth on teratomas, or an esophageal hernia, almost invariably an abnormal mediastinum noted on a chest radiograph will trigger further investigations.

Radiological Anatomic Details of the Mediastinum

The natural contrast interface between aerated lung and the mediastinum created by the low density of the air in the lungs or central airways in contrast to the higher density of the soft tissue in the mediastinal structures can be explored. In the frontal chest view, one should try to identify the superior vena cava, the margins of the right atrium, the inferior vena cava, the inferior pulmonary veins, the right paratracheal line (**Fig. 6**); the aortopulmonary window (**Fig. 7**); the azygoesophageal recess (**Fig. 8**); the anterior junction line and the anterior mediastinal triangle (**Figs. 9 and 10**); the posterior junction line (see **Fig. 9**); and the paravertebral lines (**Fig. 11**). In lateral chest view one should observe the margins of the right ventricle, the ascending aorta, the aortic arch, the posterior wall of the trachea, the posterior wall of the bronchus intermedius, the margins of the left atrium, the right and left pulmonary arteries, the pulmonary veins, the inferior vena cava, the descending aorta, and the margins of the thoracic spine (see **Fig. 5; Fig. 12**).

The anterior junction line (AJL) is only visible when the volume of fat anterior to the ascending aorta and it major branches is minimal, allowing the contact of the anterior portion of both lungs, which would be separated solely by the layers of pleurae, creating a well defined thin line or septum that extends from the upper aspect of the right ventricle up to the level of the brachiocephalic vessels, approximately at the level of the angle of Louis (angle of the sternum) (see **Figs. 9 and 10**). In the lateral view this line is not visible, but the absence of soft tissue density structures

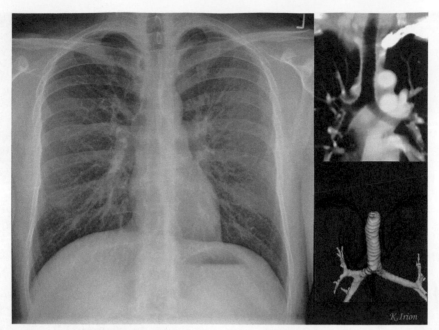

Fig. 6. Right paratracheal line and azygos vein in detail.

interposed between the lungs results in a low-density area behind the sternum and above the right ventricle, known as the retrosternal space (see **Fig. 12**). In the average-sized adult, the AJL measures approximately 5 to 8 cm in length and 2.5 cm in the AP diameter.

The posterior junction line (PJL) is also visible thanks to the contact between both lungs, separated solely by the pleurae, behind the esophagus.

This line is discontinued at the level of the aortic arch. Superiorly, the PJL extends to the level of the lung apex where it diverges and disappears (see **Fig. 9**).

Discrimination between the anterior and PJL is important because their displacement by a space-occupying process allows the disease to be localized on the standard chest radiograph. Also, the inability to see an AJL that was previously

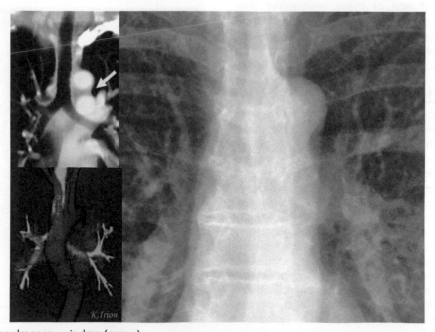

Fig. 7. Aortopulmonary window (*arrow*).

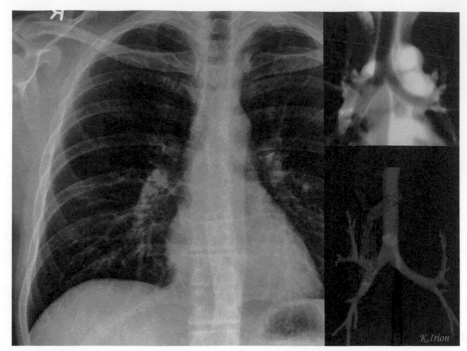

Fig. 8. The azygoesophageal recess. On the right the image was generated using thick coronal reformat from CT images, allowing the identification of the azygoesophageal recess and the azygos arch. The vertical portion of the azygos vein is parallel to the esophagus, in front of the thoracic spine, to the right of the descending aorta. Just below the level of the tracheal carina, the azygos starts to deviate its path anteriorly and toward the right to cross over the right upper lobe bronchus and drain into the superior vena cava.

visible on chest radiographs can be the initial sign of a mediastinal mass. By contrast, a well-defined AJL cannot rule out anterior mediastinal masses.

A mediastinal mass can cause displacement or annulment of one of these mediastinal lines, particularly a large anterior mediastinal mass. However, one should be aware that, not infrequently, these lines are not visible at all on chest radiographs.[7]

Paraspinal Lines

The reflection of the pleurae in the paravertebral region can frequently be identified in chest radiographs as thin lines (as thick as a normal pleura should be) running parallel to the thoracic spine, particularly in the lower zones. The paravertebral fat is responsible for the visibility of these lines, which are not always visible. The paraspinal lines can be difficult to identify in slim patients in whom the lines may closely reflect the undulations of the lateral spinal ligaments. In larger patients these undulations are smoothed out and the lines are straighter. Osteophytes, paravertebral abscesses, or vertebral metastases and schwannomas are frequent causes of deformity of these lines, which will be focally pushed away from the vertebral bodies.

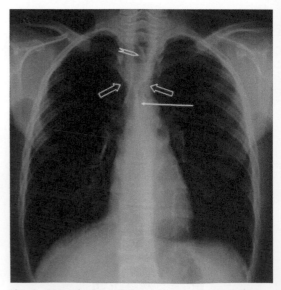

Fig. 9. Frontal view of the chest with arrows demarcating relevant anatomic details: posterior junction line (*chevron*), anterior mediastinal triangle (*open arrows*), and anterior junction line (*arrow*).

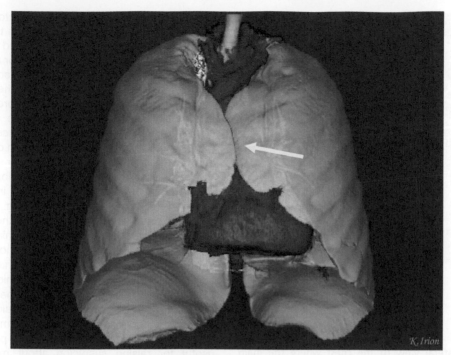

Fig. 10. Anterior mediastinal junction line (*arrow*).

Mediastinal Boundaries in Frontal Chest Radiography

Right-side mediastinum boundaries
The middle mediastinum right margins are composed by the right brachiocephalic vein, the superior vena cava, the right atrium, and the inferior vena cava (**Fig. 13**). If one accepts the mediastinal division proposed above, the posterior mediastinum right margin is given by the right paratracheal line. This line or stripe can be almost

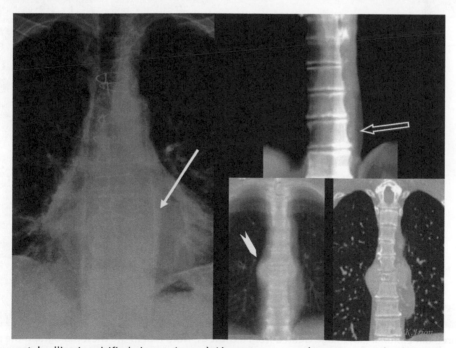

Fig. 11. Paravertebralline in calcified pleurae (*arrow*). Linear tomogram demonstrating the descending aorta and the paravertebralline behind and medial to the aorta (*open arrow*). Abnormal paravertebrallines due to bone metastasis (*chevron*).

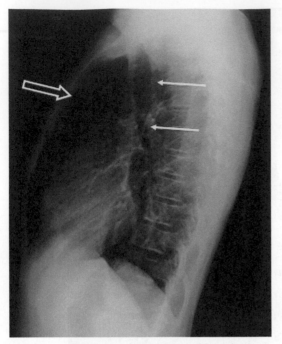

Fig. 12. Lateral view of the chest where the main anatomic repairs are being highlighted: posterior wall of the trachea and posterior wall of the bronchus intermedius (*arrows*). Retrosternal space (*open arrow*).

always identified, if the exposure factors of the radiograph are optimized to transpose the densities of the right brachiocephalic vein and the superior vena cava, which are more anterior and more towards the right than the right paratracheal line. This line represents the right wall of the trachea, which can be visible thanks to the presence of air contained in the trachea and the air in the adequately inflated lung which is adjacent to the tracheal wall, allowing the identification of its inner and outer surfaces (**Fig. 14**). The outer surface of the left wall of the trachea is not visible, as the aortic arch and its branches are interposed between the trachea and the left lung. Inferiorly, the right paratracheal line stops at the level of the azygos vein (see **Fig. 14**). The thickness of the right paratracheal line should not exceed 5 mm. It can be visible in approximately two-thirds of normal subjects. When thicker than 5 mm, one should suspect paratracheal lymphadenopathy, tracheal wall mass, right-sided aortic arch, or other less common abnormalities. In patients with lung cancer, this line is particularly useful for raising suspicion about mediastinal lymphadenopathy. In obese patients, however, this line can be thickened due to excessive mediastinal adiposity.

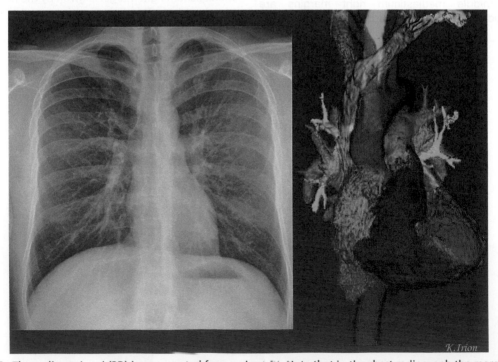

Fig. 13. Three-dimensional (3D) image created from a chest CT. Note that in the chest radiograph the margins of the middle mediastinum are given by the vessels and heart from top to bottom. On the right: right brachiocephalicvein, superior vena cava, right atrium, and inferior vena cava. On the left: left brachiocephalicvein, aortic arch, left pulmonary artery, and pulmonary trunk and left ventricle.

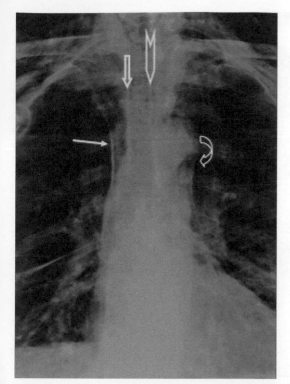

Fig. 14. Detailed chest radiograph of a patient with pneumomediastinum. The air interposed between the anatomic structures facilitates the identification of the pleural surface adjoining the superior vena cava (*arrow*) and the left wall of the trachea (*chevron*), which are not visible in the absence of pneumomediastinum. Note also the right paratracheal line (*open arrow*) and the aortopulmonary window (*curved arrow*).

Below the azygos arch, the posterior mediastinum is delimited by the reflection of the pleura in the azygoesophageal recess, which can be seen thanks to the contrast of the aerated lung contacting the soft tissue structures of the posterior mediastinum, particularly the esophagus, the azygos vein, and the descending aorta (**Fig. 15**). With an adequate degree of penetration of the x-rays, the azygoesophageal recess can be seen behind the heart shadow, extending from the diaphragm as a straight line that will divert toward the right, approximately at the level of the subcarinal region, as a consequence of the orientation of the azygos veins (azygos arch), to lying over the right main bronchus to drain into the superior vena cava (see **Fig. 6**). At the level of the subcarinal region, the azygoesophageal recess assumes a curved shape, which is almost invariably concave toward the right lung. One should suspect subcarinal lymphadenopathy, esophageal mass, or significant enlargement of the left atrium when this line is straightened or is convex toward

the right lung (see **Fig. 1**). An azygoesophageal recess which is convex towards the right lung has a high specificity for mediastinal mass, but the sensitivity for detection of subcarinal lymphadenopathy is poor (**Fig. 16**).

Left-side mediastinum boundaries

On the left side, the aortic knuckle is generally promptly recognized as a round opacity. Above the aortic arch, the left margins of the mediastinum are composed by the left carotid and subclavian arteries, and the left brachiocephalic, left jugular, and left subclavian veins (**Fig. 17**). The usual appearance on the frontal projection forms a gentle curve created by the orientation of the left subclavian artery. As mentioned earlier, the outer margin of the left tracheal wall is virtually never outlined, because the lung is separated from the trachea by the aorta and the other vessels listed above.

Immediately below the aortic knuckle, one can identify an area of lower attenuation in between the inferior aspect of the knuckle and the superior aspect of the central portion of the left pulmonary artery. This space is known as the aortopulmonary window (APW) (**Fig. 18**). The lower density of the APW is created by the presence of mediastinal fat and also by the insinuation of the left lung into this small space, which has a concave left lateral margin in the normal condition. Enlarged nodes are the most common cause of obliteration of this space, increasing its attenuation coefficients (radiological density) and deforming its concave shape, which will turn to be convex, pushing the left lung.

Distal to the APW the middle mediastinum margins are defined by the central portion of the left pulmonary artery, pulmonary trunk (main pulmonary artery), left atrium appendage, and left ventricle.

Above the level of the aortic arch, the margins of the posterior mediastinum are defined mainly by the esophagus, trachea, and paraspinal soft tissues. Below the arch, the posterior mediastinum margins are defined by the descending aorta and paraspinal tissues. The silhouette varies with the degree of tortuosity of the aorta.

Lateral Chest Radiography

The retrosternal space, which usually measures approximately 2.5 cm in the anteroposterior direction (see **Fig. 12**). Anterior mediastinal masses will insinuate in the retrosternal space between the lungs, and will increase the attenuation coefficients of this space, making this area more opaque than usual. The retrosternal space ends at the point of contact of the left ventricle with the anterior chest wall, generally at the level of the lower third of the sternum body.

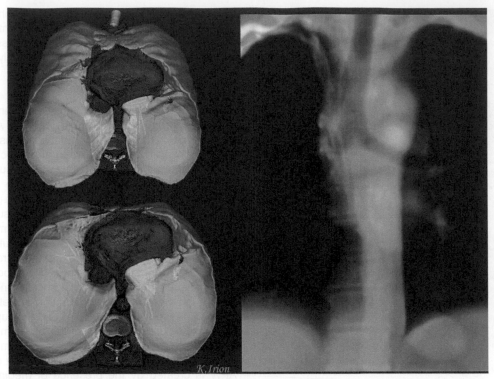

Fig. 15. Three-dimensional (3D) image created from a chest CT. Note that in the chest radiograph the margins of the middle mediastinum are given by the vessels and heart from top to bottom. On the right: right brachiocephalicvein, superior vena cava, right atrium, and inferior vena cava. On the left: left brachiocephalicvein, aortic arch, left pulmonary artery, and pulmonary trunk and left ventricle.

On some occasions, it is possible to identify a thin line internal to the sternal body, known as the retrosternal line. The retrosternal line is more commonly seen in obese patients with abundant adipose tissue separating the pleural surface from the inner surface of the sternum. The extrapleural space in this region contains internal mammary vessels, lymphatics, and intercostal

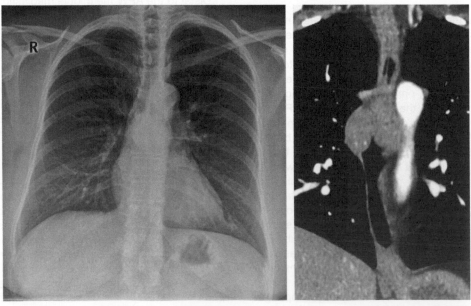

Fig. 16. Esophageal mass obliterating the azygoesophageal recess, which in this abnormal status is convex to the right lung instead of concave.

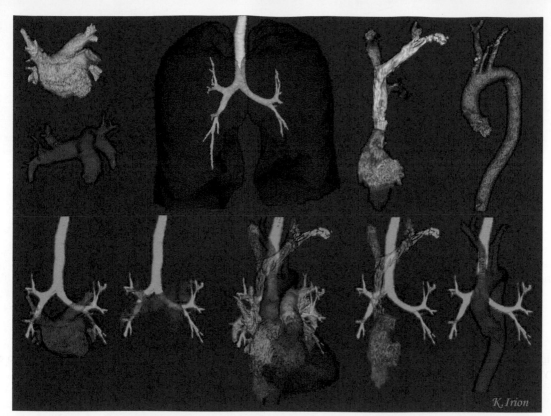

Fig. 17. 3D image showing the relation of the main vessels and the trachea. Above the aortic arch, the left margins of the mediastinum are composed by the left carotid and subclavian arteries, the left brachiocephalic, left jugular, and left subclavian veins. (Copyright K. Irion, printed with permission.)

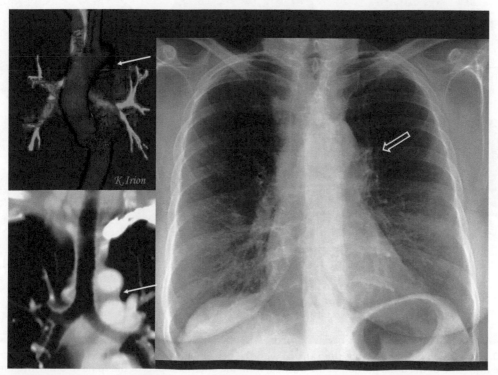

Fig. 18. 3D image showing the relation of the main vessels and the trachea. Above the aortic arch, the left margins of the mediastinum are composed by the left carotid and subclavianarteries, the left brachiocephalic, left jugular, and left subclavianveins.

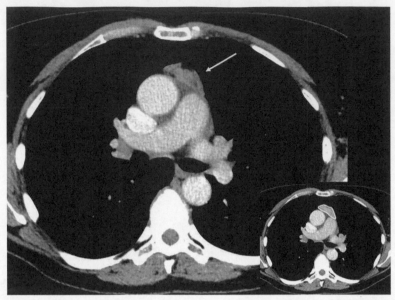

Fig. 19. Thymus in the anterior compartment: aorta and pulmonary trunk posterior and sternum anterior to a hyperplasticthymus gland.

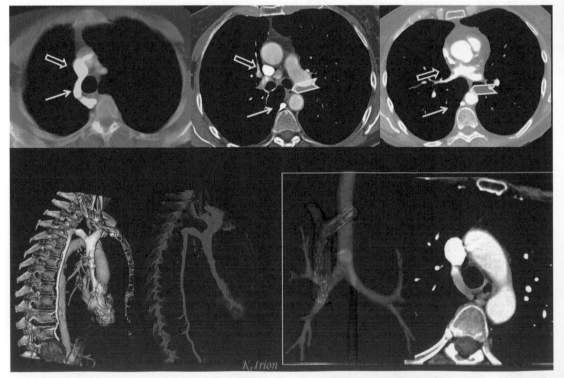

Fig. 20. Correlation between azygos (*thin arrow*) with the descending aorta and oesophagus (*chevron*), crossing on the right side of the distal portion of the trachea, from the anterior aspect of the spine to drain into the superior vena cava (*open arrow*), and azygos vein. Please note that the azygos arch is shifted upwards in this patient as a consequence of right upper lobectomy. Within the yellow box inset, the axial and the 3D reformatedimage of a patient with the azygos arch in its usual position.

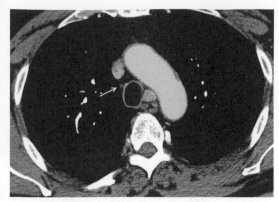

Fig. 21. Correlation between the cross of the aorta (*pink*), the superior vena cava (*blue*), and the trachea (*green*) and node (*yellow*). The arrow points the vagusnerve, which is not always visible on CT.

nerves. The retrosternal line may appear slightly undulated at the confluence of the ribs on the sternum. Enlarged nodes in the mammary nodal stations, pleural plaques or pleural masses, schwannomas, and sternum abnormalities can increase the distance between the lungs and the sternum, pushing the retrosternal line dorsally.

Frequently the retrosternal space can be partially obliterated at the level of the cardiophrenic angles, as epicardial fat pad can insinuate into this area. Sometimes this extends laterally and can simulate segmental lung collapse or even middle lobe collapse.

In the posterior mediastinum, it is possible to identify the column of air in the trachea (see **Fig. 12**). Frequently the posterior wall of the trachea is in direct contact with the aerated right upper lobe, making it possible to identify the posterior tracheal wall as a thin line (as thin as the membranous portion of the trachea should be), known as the posterior tracheal band. As the right pulmonary artery courses anterior to the right main bronchus and bronchus intermedius, it is possible to follow the line downwards, formed by the posterior walls of the right main bronchus and of the bronchus intermedius. On the left side, however, the esophagus and the aorta are interposed between the left lung and the trachea and the left pulmonary artery is interposed between the left main bronchus and left lower lobe bronchus, making it impossible to judge the thickness of the posterior wall of these segments of the airways. The esophagus will only be

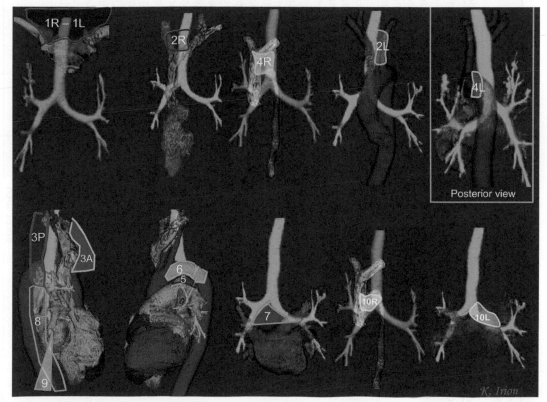

Fig. 22. Mediastinal nodal stations based on the IASLC TNM nodal map. The boundaries of each station are described in the **Table 1**. (Copyright K. Irion, printed with permission.)

Table 1
TNM 7th Edition Nodal Map

Nodal Zone	Lymph Nde Sation	Superior Margin	Inferior Margin	Right-Left Brundary
Upper zone	1R or 1L	Low cervical, supraclavicular, sternal notch	Inferior margin of crycoid cartilage	Clavicles and upper margin of the manubrium	Midline of the trachea
	2R or 2L	Upper paratracheal	Right (2R): apex of the right lung and pleural space, and in the midline, the upper border of the manubrium; Left (2L) apex of the left lung and pleural space, and in the midline, the upper border of the manubrium	Right (2R): intersection of caudal margin of innominate vein with the trachea; Left (2L) superior border of the aortic arch	Left lateral border of the trachea
	3a or 3p	Prevascular and retrotracheal (a = anterior; p = posterior)	Apex of chest; posterior aspect of sternum; 3a R: anterior border of superior vena cava; 3a L: anterior to the left carotid artery; 3p: apex of chest; posterior border of the trachea	Level of carina	Not stated
	4R or 4L	Lower paratracheal (includes nodes lateral and anterior to the trachea)	4R: intersection of caudal margin of innominate vein with the trachea; 4L: upper margin of the aortic arch; medial to the ligamentum arteriosum	4R: lower border of azygos vein; 4L: upper rim of the left main pulmonary artery	Left lateral border of the trachea
Aortopulmonary zone	5	Subaortic (aortopulmonary window)	The lower border of the aortic arch; lateral to the ligamentum arteriosum	Upper rim of the left main pulmonary artery	No division
	6	Para-aortic (ascending aorta or phrenic nerve); anterior and lateral to the ascending aorta and aortic arch	A line tangential to the upper border of the aortic arch	The lower border of the aortic arch	The boundaries between 3a and 6 is not stated

Zone	#	Node			
Subcarinal zone	7	Subcarinal	The carina of the trachea	The lower border of the bronchus intermedius on the right; the upper border of the lower lobe bronchus on the left	No division
Lower zone	8	Paraesophageal (nodes lying adjacent to the wall of the esophagus)	The lower border of the bronchus intermedius on the right; the upper border of the lower lobe bronchus on the left	The diaphragm	The midline (of the oesophagus?)
	9	Pulmonary ligament	The inferior pulmonary vein	The diaphragm	Right or left pulmonary ligaments
Hilar zone	10	Hilar (adjacent to the mainstem bronchus and hilar vessels, including the proximal portions of the pulmonary veins and main pulmonary artery)	The lower rim of the azygos vein on the right; the upper rim of the pulmonary artery on the left	Interlobar region	Right or left lung
	11s or 11i	Interlobar (s = superior; i = inferior) (between the origin of the lobar bronchi)	a#11s: between the upper lobe bronchus and bronchus intermedius on the right a#11i: between the middle and lower lobe bronchi on the right		Right or left lung
Peripheral zone	12	Lobar			
	13	Segmental			
	14	Subsegmental			

Data from Rusch V, Asamura H, Watanabe H, et al. The IASLC lung cancer staging project: a proposal for a new international lymph node map in the forthcoming seventh edition of the TNM classification for lung cancer. J Thorac Oncol 2009;4:568–77.

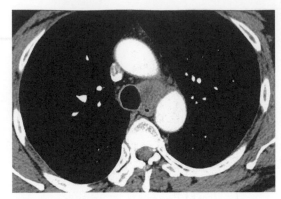

Fig. 23. Mediastinal lymphadenopathy, level 4L (*green*), highly suspicious for lung cancer. Histological samples of nodes at this level are easily obtained by endobronchial ultrasound biopsy.

identified in the lateral chest radiograph if distended with air or a significant volume of residue, or in the presence of a large esophageal mass.

COMPUTED TOMOGRAPHY
The Technique

The advent of the CT scan allowed not only a precise understanding of the normal anatomy of the mediastinum but also its correlation with abnormal processes. The better contrast resolution, characteristic of the CT images, allows the different mediastinal organs and demonstrates the lesion directly; this leads to precise localization, assessment of its extension, and its relations with neighboring organs.[2] Most masses involving the mediastinum require surgical resection. However, the choice among the various surgical approaches is dictated by the nature of the lesion as sometimes can be established based on the CT findings.[8]

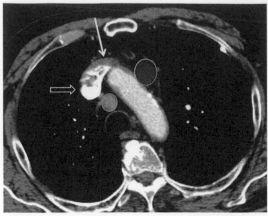

Fig. 25. Division between level 2R and 4R, inferior margin of the left brachiocephalicvein when crossing in front of the trachea and aorta. The arrow points the left brachiocephalicvein which merges with the right brachiocephalicvein to drain into the superior vena cava (*open arrow*). Node 4R (*blue*) and node 6 (*red*).

The volumetric acquisition with thin slices provided by the current CT scanners allows reconstruction of the image data in any plane with a high definition, avoiding the problem of overlapping tissues with similar densities characteristic of the chest radiographs. Also, tridimensional reconstruction, densitometric analysis, and edge enhancement algorithms offered by current CT scanners facilitate our understanding of the imaging findings. Measurements of attenuation values of a mass can provide clues for establishing the differential diagnosis. Iodinated contrast

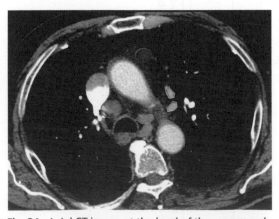

Fig. 24. Axial CT image at the level of the azygos arch. Visible nodes, some of them above the threshold of 1cm in the shortest diameter. Levels 4R (*blue*), 4L (*green*), 5 (*yellow*) and 6 (*red*).

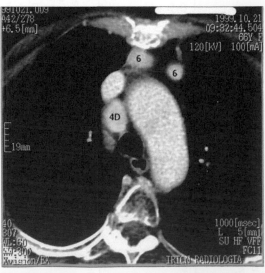

Fig. 26. Anterior mediastinal lymphadenopathy (6) and right paratracheal lymphadenopathy (4D).

material can help significantly by demonstrating the lumen and walls of vascular structures and by demonstrating areas of necrosis within solid lesions. Different enhancing patters of some lesions can also help in differentiating some types of mediastinal masses, especially thyroid masses and mediastinal cysts. Preferably intravenous contrast medium should be administered unless there are contraindications.

Density in particular is extremely important. Mediastinal masses may have low, high, or fat attenuation. Low-attenuation lesions have higher density than fat but lower than muscle, whereas high attenuation indicates a density higher than that of muscle. Conditions such as mediastinal lipomatosis, or lesions such as thymolipoma, teratoma, lipoma, and liposarcoma, can contain pockets of fat or fat tissue can be the predominant or the predominant component of a mediastinal mass. Low-attenuation lesions are generally cystic or a mass may show low attenuation when containing cystic/necrotic areas, such as in cystic

thymoma, germ-cell tumors, lymphangioma and hemangioma, mediastinal abscesses, hematoma, and primary or necrotic tumors. Examples of high-density masses include calcific lymphadenopathy as in granulomatous infections, sarcoidosis, silicosis, adenocarcinoma and sarcoma metastasis, treated lymphoma, partially calcific and primary tumors (germ-cell tumors, thymoma), and mediastinal hematoma.

Mediastinal Anatomy on CT

The thymus is situated anterior to the aorta and pulmonary artery, for the most part in the anterior mediastinum sometimes extending into the neck (**Fig. 19**). The thymus is often best seen on a coronal section through the aortic arch or great vessels.[9] Before puberty the thymus occupies most of the anterior mediastinum, between the great vessels and the anterior chest wall as if molded by these structures. In adults the thymus is bilobed or triangular in shape, but approximate

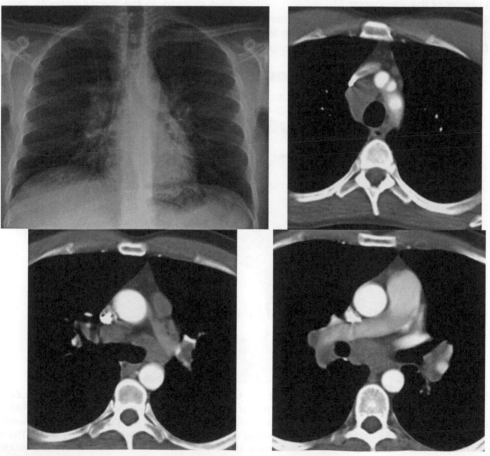

Fig. 27. Mediastinal lymphadenopathy. Correlation of the plain radiograph obliteration of the right paratracheal region, aortopulmonary window, and subcarinal region with the CT scan images showing enlarged nodes in the stations 2R, 3, 4R, 4L, 5, 6, 7, 10R and 10 L.

symmetry is the rule.[10] Between the ages of 20 and 50 years the average thickness, as measured by CT, decreases from 8 to 9 mm to 5 to 6 mm, the maximum thickness of each lobe being up to 15 mm in length.[11]

In younger patients, the CT density of the thymus is homogeneous and shows attenuation values close to that of other soft tissues.[12] After puberty this density gradually decreases due to fatty replacement. For those older than 40 years the thymus usually has an attenuation value similar to the adjacent mediastinal fat.[10,11]

The trachea lies as an immediate anterior relation of the thoracic esophagus, which itself lies immediately in front of the upper thoracic vertebral bodies (**Figs. 20** and **21**). The right vagus descends through the superior mediastinum closely applied to the right border of the trachea. The vagus then passes behind the right pulmonary hilum to reach the esophagus. The thoracic duct ascends along the right side of the esophagus, passes obliquely behind it at the level of T5, and then, in the superior mediastinum, ascends along the left border of the esophagus.

Lymph nodes are widely distributed in the mediastinum (**Fig. 22**). The absolute majority are less than 10 mm in diameter, and only few exceptions have a diameter less than 15 mm.[13,14] When enlarged, nodes should be regarded as abnormal, either due to an inflammatory process or a neoplastic process (**Fig. 23**). Enlarged nodes can also be found in patients with cardiac failure and pleural effusion, engorged by the fluid overload. In the paraspinal areas, in the region of the brachiocephalic veins (see **Fig. 29**), and in the space behind the diaphragmatic crura, lymph nodes are in general smaller, 6 mm or less, whereas nodes in the aortopulmonary window (**Fig. 24**), paratracheal space can measure between 6 and 10 mm (shortest diameter) (**Figs. 25** and **26**). Normal nodes in the subcarinal compartment (**Fig. 27**) can measure up to 12 mm in the shortest diameter.[14,15]

A structure is radiologically defined as a mediastinal lymph node if it has a soft tissue density, well defined margins, is round or oval in shape and is readily distinguished from vascular or neurogenic structures. The presence of mediastinal fat greatly facilitates the CT depiction of lymph nodes. When calcified, the nodes are promptly visible and usually calcification indicates a prior granulomatous disease. In the normal patients, mediastinal nodes are more commonly seen in the regions close to the trachea, the main bronchi, posterior to the innominate (left brachiocephalic) vein and

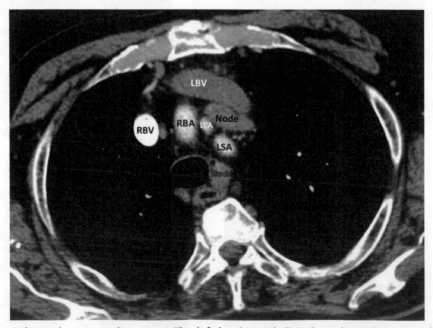

Fig. 28. Prevascular and retrovascular spaces. The left brachiocephalic vein or innominate vein (LBV) courses downwards and to the right, in front of the right brachiocephalic artery or innominate artery (RBA) to join the right brachiocephalic vein (RBV) to form the superior vena cava. Note the presence of an abnormal node interposed between the LBV and the left carotid artery (LCA) and the left subclavian artery (LSA). The space in front of the LBV was also known as pre-innominate space and the space behind this vessel was known as retro-innominate space. This distinction should be avoided, as it may create confusion in the localization of mediastinal nodes. The node interposed between the LBV and the LSA is regarded as in the level 3, despite being in the retro-innominate space.

between the aorta and the left pulmonary artery (see **Figs. 25–27**).

A nodal map had been developed to localize the mediastinal nodes.[16] Since 2009, the nodal map proposed by Mountain and Dressler and adopted by the AJCC-UICC has been replaced by a new map developed by Rusch et al on behalf of the IASLC (**Fig. 22**).[16,17]

Prevascular and Retrovascular Spaces

The left innominate vein courses downward and to the right in front of the innominate artery to join with the right innominate vein, forming the superior vena cava (**Fig. 28**). The left brachiocephalic vein is the main structure which defines the boundaries between the pre-vascular and retrovascular spaces.

Pretracheal Space

The space previously known as the pretracheal space or right tracheobronchial angle is bounded by the superior vena cava anteriorly, the trachea posteriorly, the ascending aorta on the left, and the azygos arch on the right (**Fig. 29**).[18] This term pretracheal space should be avoided as it cannot be used for localizing mediastinal nodes, which should be identified as per the new Nodal Map described above.

Subcarinal Space

The subcarinal space is bounded by: the right pulmonary artery, the left superior pulmonary

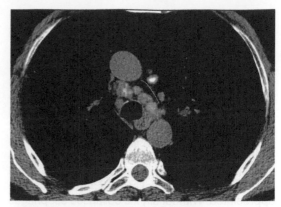

Fig. 30. Aortopulmonary window and left lower paratracheal regions divided by the ligamentum arteriosum (*yellow line*).

vein and the left atrium anteriorly, the esophagus, azygos vein and aorta posteriorly, right and left-lower-lobe mediastinal pleurae laterally (see **Fig. 27**). The boundaries of this space also cannot be used for localizing mediastinal nodes, which should be identified as per the new Nodal Map described above.

Aortopulmonary Window

The boundaries include the ascending aorta anteriorly, the descending aorta posteriorly, the ligamentum arteriosum medially, the left upper-lobe

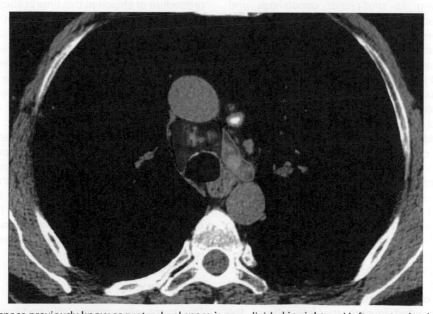

Fig. 29. The space previously know as pretracheal space is now divided in right and left paratracheal regions. The nodes within the area demarcated in red are right paratracheal nodes and the nodes within the area demarcated in green are left paratracheal nodes. Lateral to the ligamentum arteriosum lye the aortopulmonary window nodes.

pleurae laterally, the aortic arch superiorly, and the left pulmonary artery inferiorly (see **Fig. 26; Fig. 30**).

Esophagus

The esophagus is visible on all axial CT and MRI sections from the root of the neck down to the diaphragm (see **Fig. 20**). It may contain a small amount of air in approximately 80% of normal people. If there is sufficient mediastinal fat, the entire circumference of the esophagus can be identified, and if air is present in the esophageal lumen, the uniform thickness of the wall can be appreciated. Without air, the collapsed esophagus appears circular or oval in shape and measures approximately 1 cm in its narrowest diameter.[19] The esophagus is discussed in detail in another article by Ugalde and colleagues elsewhere in this issue.

MAGNETIC RESONANCE IMAGING

MRI has not been as extensively used as CT in the study of chest pathology. The reason is that it has suffered from certain technical limitations—mainly artifacts caused by respiratory and cardiac movements—but technological progress has made gating systems available and has allowed the acquisition of fast sequences that are virtually free of artifacts and are used in cardiovascular imaging.[20] Also, its use is more limited in the assessment of diseases of the lung parenchyma.

Considering its multiplanar capabilities and excellent depiction of musculoskeletal structures, MRI is generally suitable for studying processes located near the lung apex and spine and in the chest wall, as well as disorders of the mediastinal vessels and peridiaphragmatic regions. Moreover, its high capacity for tissue differentiation allows discrimination, in a single examination, between pleural involvement and parenchymal consolidation and mediastinal and chest wall involvement.[21]

The lack of ionizing radiation, the ability to do multiplanar imaging, and the unnecessary intravenous contrast media in assessing thoracic vascular structures makes MRI an attractive alternative to CT scanning in the thorax.[22] Moreover, compared with CT, MRI has the advantage that contrast material can also be administered to patients with impaired renal function. Its limitations, on the other hand, are claustrophobia, compliance of debilitated patients, examination times, high cost, and limited availability.

In T1-weighted images the intensity of the esophagus is similar to that of muscle and appreciably lower than that of mediastinal fat, although, as would be expected, this difference decreases with age. On T2-weighted images, the intensity differences are slight and do not vary with age. On MR scans, the esophagus may be mistaken for an enlarged retrotracheal lymph node on a single image. The signal intensity on T1-weighted images is similar to muscle but on T2-weighted images the esophagus often shows much higher signal intensity than muscle.[19]

Scattered calcifications within enlarged mediastinal and hilar lymph nodes due to old granulomatous disease are not detectable by MRI.[23] Small calcifications may have no signal or low signal intensity and may lead to an interpretation of inhomogeneous signal intensity lymphadenopathy.

Many patients are unsuitable for MR scanning. Seriously ill patients cannot be monitored and managed adequately. Patients with pacemakers or certain ferromagnetic vascular surgical clips also may not be scanned. The limitations of MRI in evaluating the mediastinum in bronchogenic carcinoma also apply to the evaluation of other mediastinal and/or hilar masses.[22,24] In particular, discrete clustered normal-sized lymph nodes may appear as a single large lymph node mass on MRI, and calcified hilar lymph nodes may also be misinterpreted as adenopathy of unknown cause.[23] MRI probably should be reserved for cases in which intravenous contrast material is contraindicated or where postcontrast CT scans are inconclusive.[22] Because of the requirement for patient selection and the pitfalls of MRI within the mediastinum, the authors believe CT remains the radiologic procedure of choice at this time in staging patients with bronchogenic carcinoma and other mediastinal and/or hilar masses.[2,13,24]

Indications for MRI are therefore limited: it may be used as a third-level investigation to complement CT but not as a routine study. MRI has proved superior to CT in selected cases only: assessment of vascular lesions; definition of vascular involvement by extrinsic pathologic processes; study of the chest wall and posterior mediastinum; imaging of the paravertebral regions, nerve plexuses and neurogenic tumors; recognition, within the mediastinal structures and heart, cleavage planes and their invasion by tumors, particularly when the CT findings are doubtful; and differential diagnosis between fibrous tissue and persistence or recurrence of neoplasm after radiation therapy.

SUMMARY

Due to the easy accessibility and low cost, chest radiography continues to be the standard initial workup of intrathoracic disorders. Recently, digital radiography added little to improve the sensitivity and specificity of the conventional chest radiograph; however, the quality of the image has indeed increased. Because only the boundary between the lung and the mediastinal structures are visualized, plain chest radiographs provide limited information regarding mediastinal anatomy. CT has become the standard technique to evaluate the mediastinum, and is also the radiologic procedure of choice for staging bronchogenic carcinoma and determining the solid or vascular nature and extent of other mediastinal and/or hilar masses. Where MRI provides the same diagnostic information as CT, CT should be preferred. The elective role of MRI remains limited to the study of the cardiovascular system.

REFERENCES

1. Priola SM, Priola AM, Cardinale L, et al. The anterior mediastinum: anatomy and imaging procedures. Radiol Med 2006;111(3):295–311.
2. Epstein DM, Kressel H, Gefter W, et al. MR imaging of the mediastinum: a retrospective comparison with computed tomography. J Comput Assist Tomogr 1984;8(4):670–6.
3. Gamsu G, Webb WR, Sheldon P, et al. Nuclear magnetic resonance imaging of the thorax. Radiology 1983;147(2):473–80.
4. Hansell DM, Bankier AA, MacMahon H, et al. Fleischner Society: glossary of terms for thoracic imaging. Radiology 2008;246(3):697–722.
5. MacMahon H, Doi K. Digital chest radiography. Clin Chest Med 1991;12(1):19–32.
6. Foley WD, Lawson TL, Scanlon GT, et al. Digital radiograph of the chest using a computed tomography instrument. Radiology 1979;133(1):231–4.
7. Gibbs JM, Chandrasekhar CA, Ferguson EC, et al. Lines and stripes: where did they go?—From conventional radiography to CT. Radiographics 2007;27(1):33–48.
8. Zylak CJ, Pallie W, Jackson R. Correlative anatomy and computed tomography: a module on the mediastinum. Radiographics 1982;2(4):555–92.
9. Mendelson DS. Imaging of the thymus. Chest Surg Clin N Am 2001;11(2):269–93.
10. Baron RL, Lee JK, Sagel SS, et al. Computed tomography of the normal thymus. Radiology 1982;142(1):121–5.
11. Dixon AK, Hilton CJ, Williams CT. Computed tomography and histological correlation of the thymic remnant. Clin Radiol 1981;32(3):255–7.
12. Moore AV, Korobkin M, Olanow W, et al. Age-related changes in the thymus gland: CT-pathologic correlation. AJR Am J Roentgenol 1983;141(2):241–6.
13. Faling LJ, Pugatch RD, Jung-Legg Y, et al. Computed tomographic scanning of the mediastinum in the staging of bronchogenic carcinoma. Am Rev Respir Dis 1981;124(6):690–5.
14. Ingram CE, Belli AM, Lewars MD, et al. Normal lymph node size in the mediastinum: a retrospective study in two patient groups. Clin Radiol 1989;40(1):35–9.
15. Genereux GP, Howie JL. Normal mediastinal lymph node size and number: CT and anatomic study. AJR Am J Roentgenol 1984;142(6):1095–100.
16. Rusch VW, Asamura H, Watanabe H, et al. The IASLC lung cancer staging project: a proposal for a new international lymph node map in the forthcoming seventh edition of the TNM classification for lung cancer. J Thorac Oncol 2009;4(5):568–77.
17. Rusch VW, Crowley J, Giroux DJ, et al. The IASLC lung cancer project: proposals for the revision of the N descriptors in the forthcoming seventh edition of the TNM classification for lung cancer. J Thorac Oncol 2007;2:603–12.
18. Schynder PA, Gamsu G. CT of the pretracheal retrocaval space. AJR Am J Roentgenol 1981;136(2):303–8.
19. Riddell AM, Davies DC, Allum WH, et al. High-resolution MRI in evaluation of the surgical anatomy of the esophagus and posterior mediastinum. AJR Am J Roentgenol 2007;188(1):W37–43.
20. Aunge VM, Clanton JA, Partain CL, et al. Respiratory gating in magnetic resonance imaging at 0.5 tesla. Radiology 1984;151(2):521–3.
21. O'Donovan PB, Ross JS, Sivak ED, et al. Magnetic resonance imaging of the thorax: the advantages of coronal and sagittal planes. AJR Am J Roentgenol 1984;143(6):1183–8.
22. Cohen AM, Creviston S, LiPuma JP, et al. Nuclear magnetic resonance imaging of the mediastinum and hili: early impressions of its efficacy. AJR Am J Roentgenol 1983;141(6):1163–9.
23. Levitt RG, Glazer HS, Roper CL, et al. Magnetic resonance imaging of mediastinal and hilar masses: comparison with CT. AJR Am J Roentgenol 1985;145(1):9–14.
24. Webb WA, Gamsu G, Stark DD, et al. Evaluation of magnetic resonance sequences in imaging mediastinal tumors. AJR Am J Roentgenol 1984;143(4):723–7.

FURTHER READINGS

Heitzman ER. The mediastinum. St Louis (MO): Mosby; 1977. p. 39–42.

Moore KL, Dalley FD. Clinically oriented anatomy. 5th edition. Philadelphia: Lippincott Williams and Wilkins; 2006.

Park DR, Vallières E. The normal mediastinum. In: Mason RJ, Murray JF, Broaddus VC, et al, editors.

Murray & Nadel's textbook of respiratory medicine. 4th edition. Philadelphia: Saunders; 2005.

Standing S, editor. Gray's anatomy. 39th edition. London: Elsevier; 2005.

Varghese TK Jr, Lau CL. The mediastinum. In: Townsend C Jr, Beauchamp RD, Evers BM, et al, editors. Sabiston textbook of surgery: the biological basis of modern surgical practice. 18th edition. Philadelphia: Saunders Elsevier; 2008.

Warren HW. Anatomy of the mediastinum with special reference to surgical access. In: Patterson GA, Cooper JD, Deslauriers J, et al, editors. Pearson's thoracic and esophageal surgery. 3rd edition. Philadelphia: Churchill Livingstone; 2008.

Anatomy of the Normal Diaphragm

Robert Downey, MD

KEYWORDS
- Diaphragm • Phrenic nerve • Hiatus • Embryology
- Phrenic artery • Central aponeurosis

The thoracic diaphragm is a dome-shaped septum, composed of muscle surrounding a central tendon (the central aponeurosis), which separates the thoracic and abdominal cavities. The function of the diaphragm is twofold: to expand the chest cavity during inspiration to cause air to enter the chest, and to promote occlusion of the gastroesophageal junction during inspiration to prevent reflux from the stomach into the esophagus. Given that it is a muscular structure, its biologic action is relatively simple, and the physiology and pathophysiology of the diaphragm are readily understood from the anatomic structure. This article provides an overview of the normal anatomy of the diaphragm.

EMBRYOLOGY OF THE DIAPHRAGM

The diaphragm originates from 4 portions of the developing embryo: the septum transversum from the ventral portion, 2 pleuroperitoneal folds arising laterally, and the dorsal mesentery (**Fig. 1**).[1] The septum transversum grows dorsally from the ventral body wall during the third to eighth week of gestation, providing the area of the diaphragm eventually apposed to the pericardial sac. Muscle fibers along with the neural structures that will form the phrenic nerves migrate from the third to fifth myotomes to lie between the membranes of the septum transversum and the pleuroperitoneal folds. The dorsal mesentery encompasses the developing vasculature and the digestive tract. Failure of closure between these portions can lead to residual defects. For example, a foramen of Bochdalek hernia can arise from failure of the pleuroperitoneal membrane to form a common aponeurosis with the developing

transversus abdominis between what will become the tip of the 12th rib and the quadratus lumborum. Diaphragmatic hernias occurring because of a failure of fusion of the membranes will give rise to a hernia without a sac. If the membranes fuse but the muscle fibers fail to migrate from the cervical myotomes, a hernia with a sac results.

NORMAL ANATOMY OF THE DIAPHRAGM
Muscular and Tendinous Portions of the Diaphragm Including Attachments to Surrounding Structures

The central aponeurosis of the diaphragm has been considered to have the shape of a clover leaf, with 1 anterior and 2 lateral leaves. The muscular portions attach to the central aponeurosis and to the circumference of the thoracic inlet—the ribs, the sternum, and the lumbar spine. There are 3 parts to the muscular portion of the diaphragm separated by areas without muscle—the lumbar, the costal, and the sternal—each of which insert into the central aponeurosis of the diaphragm (**Fig. 2**). On a chest radiograph, the diaphragm has the appearance of a saddle that may be caused by the upward pressure from the liver laterally and from downward pressure from the heart centrally.

The muscular portions of the diaphragm are continuous with the transversus abdominis of the abdominal wall. A subcostal incision with division of the external and internal oblique muscles of the abdominal wall along with their attachments to the costal margin will reveal that the diaphragm and the transversus abdominis form a continuous sheet with the lumbar fascia and the rectus sheath, surrounding the abdominal cavity. In other words, the diaphragm forms a continuous structure with the inner layer of the abdominal wall.[2]

Thoracic Service, Department of Surgery, Memorial Sloan-Kettering Cancer Center, 1275 York Avenue, C-871, New York, NY 10065, USA
E-mail address: downeyr@mskcc.org

Thorac Surg Clin 21 (2011) 273–279
doi:10.1016/j.thorsurg.2011.01.001

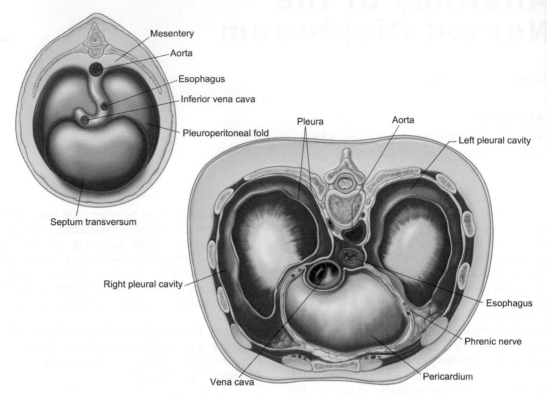

Fig. 1. Embryologic components of the diaphragm.

The sternal portion of the diaphragm is the smallest, extending from the posterior layer of the rectus sheath and from the back of the xiphoid to the central tendon of the diaphragm. Lateral to the sternal portion of the diaphragm are the costal portions, and between these portions of the diaphragm lie areas covered only by connective tissue. On one side is the right sternocostal triangle of Morgani and on the other is the left sternocostal triangle of Larrey.

The lumbar portion of the diaphragm is located on either side of the vertebral column, where the right and left crura of the diaphragm form. The relative contributions of the right and left crura to the formation of the esophageal hiatus are discussed further in a subsequent section.

Along with the transversus abdominis muscle, the costal portion of the diaphragm arises from ribs 7 to 12. Often, an area is found between the muscles of the lumbar and the costal portions of the diaphragm that is covered only by fascia. This area is called Bochdalek's gap

Blood Supply of the Diaphragm

The primary blood supply to the diaphragm enters on the inferior surface. The inferior phrenic arteries

arise from the aorta at the aortic hiatus or below to the level of or from the celiac trunk. The right phrenic artery rarely arises from the right renal artery. The inferior phrenic often divides posteriorly. A smaller branch has collateral anastomoses with branches of the 8th to 12th intercostal arteries. The larger division of the inferior phrenic artery runs anteriorly around the margin of the central tendon to form collateral anastomoses anteriorly with the pericardiophrenic and the musculophrenic arteries. The pericardiophrenic artery arises from the internal mammary artery, and accompanies the phrenic nerve on its course to the diaphragm. The musculophrenic artery also arises from the internal mammary artery, then gives off branches to the seventh to ninth intercostal spaces, as well as branches to the diaphragm anteriorly. The venous drainage of the diaphragm (the right and left inferior phrenic veins) follows the arterial supply to drain into the vena cava.

Lymphatic System of the Diaphragm

The lymphatic drainage of the diaphragm has been held to consist of 3 groups of lymph nodes. The anterior group is located adjacent to the xiphoid

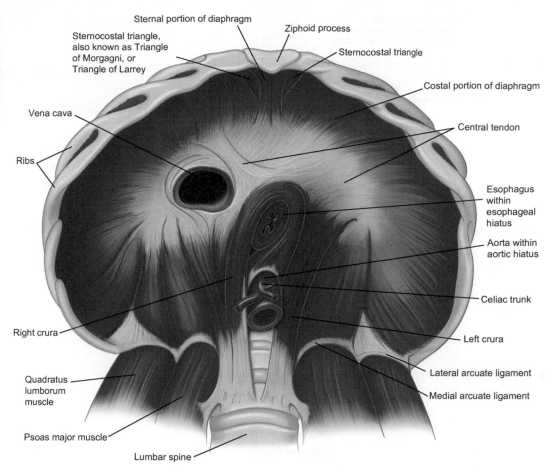

Fig. 2. Abdominal view showing the lumbar, costal, and sternal portions of the muscular diaphragm.

process. The right and left lateral group is located near to the entrance point of the phrenic nerve to the diaphragm. The posterior group is located around the diaphragmatic crura.

Openings in the Diaphragm

There are multiple openings in the diaphragm to allow passage of structures between the thoracic and abdominal cavities (**Fig. 3**).

The hiatus esophagus allows passage of the esophagus, as well as the anterior and posterior vagal trunks. The anatomy of esophageal hiatus was described in detail by Collis and colleagues.[3] The posterior aspect is formed by the median arcuate ligament. Dissection of 64 autopsy specimens without known diaphragmatic pathology suggested that in approximately 50%, there was a large right crus that provided all the structures of the esophageal hiatus, with no contribution from the left crus. In these cases, no decussation of muscle fibers of the right crus was seen, but

rather varying degrees of muscle overlap were noted. Fibers from the extreme left of the right crus cross over to form the right margin of the hiatus, and conversely, fibers from the extreme right of the left crus cross over to the right to form the left margin of the hiatus. Collis and colleagues suggest an analogy to a double-breasted coat (**Fig. 4**). In about 16% of cases, some minor contribution of the left crus to the formation of the right margin of the hiatus is seen. In the remaining third of cases, definite participation of the left crus to the formation of the right margin is seen (**Fig. 5**). Two specific individual muscle bands have been identified. The muscle of Low[4] is approximately 10 to 15 mm in width, and extends from the medial aspect of the left crus, lies on the upper surface of the diaphragm, crossing over in front of the aortic hiatus through the fibers of the right crus to end in the orifice of the inferior vena cava (**Fig. 6**). The transverse intertendinous muscle also lies on the superior surface of the diaphragm, arises from

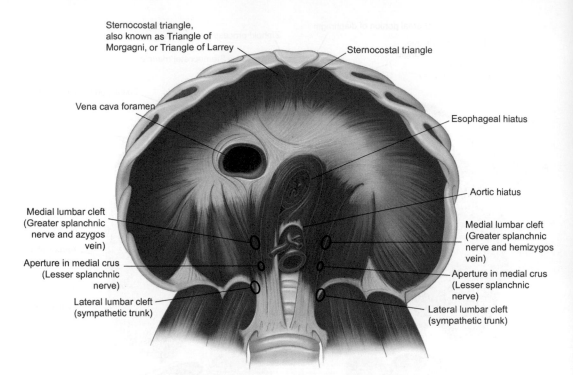

Sternocostal triangle,
also known as Triangle of
Morgagni, or Triangle of Larrey

Sternocostal triangle

Vena cava foramen

Esophageal hiatus

Aortic hiatus

Medial lumbar cleft
(Greater splanchnic
nerve and azygos
vein)

Medial lumbar cleft
(Greater splanchnic
nerve and hemizygos
vein)

Aperture in medial crus
(Lesser splanchnic
nerve)

Aperture in medial crus
(Lesser splanchnic
nerve)

Lateral lumbar cleft
(sympathetic trunk)

Lateral lumbar cleft
(sympathetic trunk)

Fig. 3. Abdominal view of the apertures through the diaphragm.

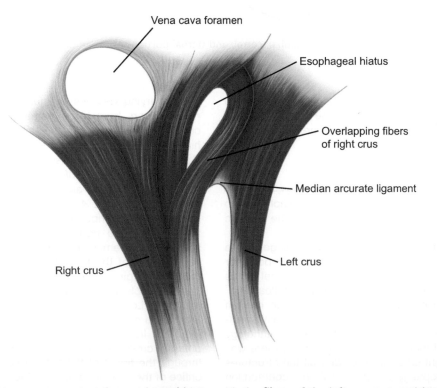

Vena cava foramen

Esophageal hiatus

Overlapping fibers
of right crus

Median arcurate ligament

Left crus

Right crus

Fig. 4. Muscular arrangement at the esophageal hiatus with the fibers of the left crus not participating in the esophageal orifice.

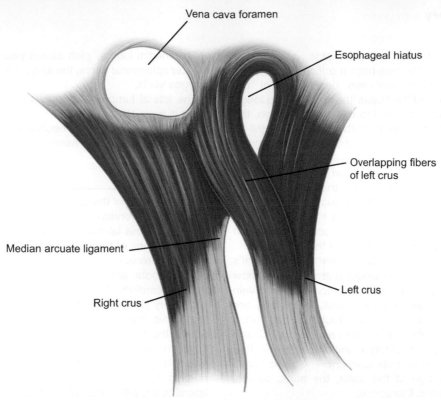

Fig. 5. Muscular arrangement at the esophageal hiatus with the fibers of the left crus participating in the esophageal orifice.

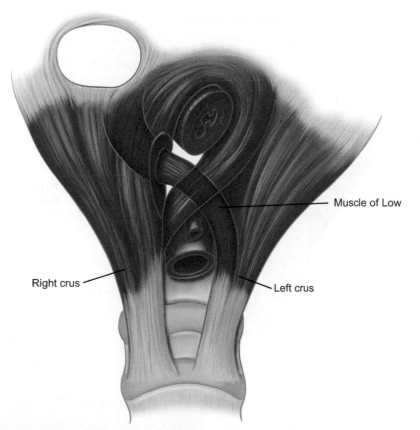

Fig. 6. Muscular arrangement at the esophageal hiatus demonstrating the muscle of Low.

the central tendon on each side, and passes posteriorly to the esophageal orifice (**Fig. 7**). The author suggests that this distribution of the muscles around the hiatus (the crus forming longitudinal bands attached to the central tendon, the crossing of muscles from the left to the right as the left contributes to the right margin, the muscle of Low, and the intertendinous muscle) works in 2 ways to maintain closure of the hiatus during inspiration. The crus keeps the angle between the esophagus and the hiatus from widening during descent, while at the same time contraction of the crossing muscles has a scissor effect that works to close the lower end of the esophagus.

The trigonum sternocostale dextrum (Morgagni's gap) and the sternocostale (Larrey's gap) allow passage of the internal mammary artery and vein into the anterior abdominal wall, where they are known as the superior epigastric artery and vein.

The aortic hiatus is located anterior to T12 and the crus of the diaphragm, and anteriorly is limited by the median arcuate ligament. The aortic hiatus allows passage of the aorta, the aortic plexus, and the ductus thoracicus.

The foramen vena cava allows passage of the inferior vena cava and the right phrenic nerve.

The medial lumbar cleft allows passage of the greater splanchnic nerve, the azygos and the hemiazygos veins.

The lateral lumbar cleft allows passage of the truncus sympathicus.

The aperture in the crus mediale allows passage of the lesser splanchnic nerve.

Nerve Supply

The innervation of the diaphragm is primarily from the phrenic nerves, although some innervation arises from the lateral diaphragm and may arise from branches of the intercostal nerves. The right and left phrenic nerves arise from the third to fifth cervical roots, and pass on the lateral surface of the pericardium to reach the diaphragm. An accessory phrenic nerve arising from the subclavian nerve may be found. The right phrenic nerve enters the central tendon directly lateral to the foramen vena cava, and from there enters the muscular portion of the diaphragm. The left phrenic nerve enters the central tendon directly lateral to the left border of the heart.

The phrenic nerve passes partially through the muscular portions of the diaphragm and so is not

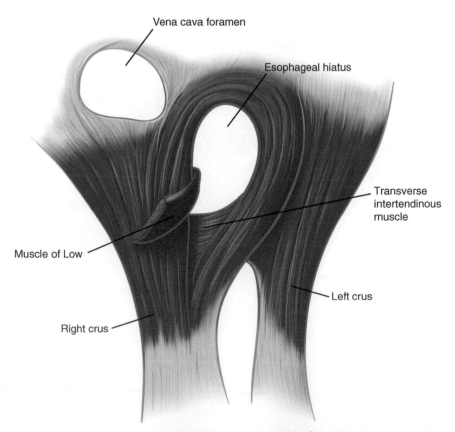

Fig. 7. Muscular arrangement at the esophageal hiatus demonstrating the transverse intertendinous muscle.

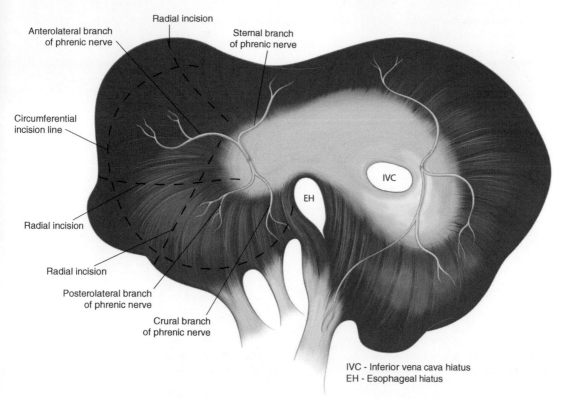

Radial incision

Anterolateral branch
of phrenic nerve

Sternal branch
of phrenic nerve

Circumferential
incision line

IVC

EH

Radial incision

Radial incision

Posterolateral branch
of phrenic nerve

Crural branch
of phrenic nerve

IVC - Inferior vena cava hiatus
EH - Esophageal hiatus

Fig. 8. Thoracic view of the diaphragm demonstrating distribution of the branches of the phrenic nerves and possible incisions.

often visible on the surface. The right and left phrenic nerves form 4 motor branches: the sternal, the anterolateral, the posterolateral, and the crural. Incisions in the diaphragm intended to avoid the phrenic nerve can be placed circumferentially several centimeters from the costal attachment. Alternatively, the incision can be placed radially between the primary motor branches, with probably the safest of these being placed between the pericardial attachment to the diaphragm and the entrance of the phrenic nerve into the diaphragm (**Fig. 8**).[5]

REFERENCES

1. Schumpelick V, Steinau G, Schluper I, et al. Surgical embryology and anatomy of the diaphragm with surgical applications. Surg Clin North Am 2000; 80(1):213–39.

2. Rives JD, Baker DD. Anatomy of the attachments of the diaphragm: their relation to the problems of the surgery of diaphragmatic hernia. Ann Surg 1942; 115(5):745–55.

3. Collis JL, Kelly TD, Wiley AM. Anatomy of the crura of the diaphragm and the surgery of hiatus hernia. Thorax 1954;9(3):175–89.

4. Low A. A note on the crura of the diaphragm and the muscle of Treitz. J Anat Physiol 1907;42(Pt 1): 93–6.

5. Merendino KA, Johnson RJ, Skinner HH, et al. The intradiaphragmatic distribution of the phrenic nerve with particular reference to the placement of diaphragmatic incisions and controlled segmental paralysis. Surgery 1956;39(1):189–98.

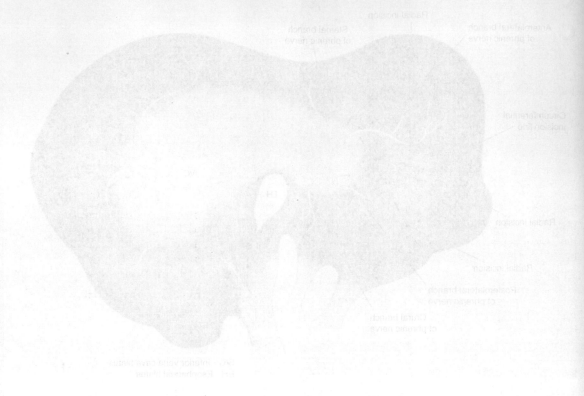

Fig. 8. The mesh view of the diaphragm demonstrating distribution of the branches of the phrenic nerves and possible incisions

Correlative Anatomy of the Diaphragm

Cao Dianbo, MD[a], Liu Wei, MD[b], Jean-Philippe Bolduc, MD[c],
Jean Deslauriers, MD, FRCS(C)[d],*

KEYWORDS

• Diaphragm • Anatomy • Imaging modalities

The diaphragm acts as a partition between the thoracic and abdominal cavities. It is covered by the parietal pleural above and the peritoneum below. The diaphragm consists of a central tendon and dome-shaped right and left leaflets made of striated muscle,[1–3] and also has lumbar and costal parts. The central tendon, which is a thin aponeurosis formed by closely interwoven fascial fibers, has the general shape of a boomerang.

On standard chest radiographs, the right hemidiaphragm is generally 1 to 2 cm higher than the left. On fluoroscopy, which is the primary means of evaluating diaphragmatic motion,[3] the diaphragm moves downward with inspiration and upward with expiration, with an average excursion of 3 to 5 cm. On computed tomography (CT) scan, the diaphragm is seen as a curved soft-tissue density with fat below and aerated lung above.[4,5] The direct multiplanar capability of magnetic resonance (MR) technology can improve depiction of normal or abnormal diaphragmatic anatomy.[6]

Despite the usefulness of these imaging modalities, adequate visualization of the diaphragm can be difficult because it is thin, has a domed contour, and is contiguous with soft tissues of the abdomen. In addition, its gross morphology and relative position can be modified by mechanical forces acting from the pleural space or abdominal cavities.[1] Despite these difficulties, each thoracic surgeon must be familiar with the correlative anatomy of the diaphragm because this knowledge is a prerequisite to making an accurate diagnosis of diaphragmatic abnormalities.

OVERALL CONFIGURATION OF THE DIAPHRAGM

The mature diaphragm consists of peripheral striated muscle fibers that converge onto a boomerang-shaped central tendon. The midportion of this central tendon fuses with the caudal aspect of the pericardium while the right and left lateral leaflets form the hemidiaphragmatic domes that are best seen on posteroanterior chest films (**Fig. 1**). The right hemidiaphragm dome usually projects at the level of the anterior sixth rib and posterior tenth rib while the left hemidiaphragm is positioned 1 or 2 cm below the right hemidiaphragm.[2,3,7] It is important to remember that the configuration and position of each hemidiaphragm is influenced not only by the pressures within the pleural spaces and peritoneal cavity but also by pathologic processes such as atelectasis, pleural effusion, and ascites that may alter those pressures. The normal diaphragm can finally have anatomic variations such as scalloped or arcuate contours, partial eventration (**Fig. 2**), or hypertrophic crus, which have usually no or little clinical relevance.

[a] Department of Radiology, First Teaching Hospital of Jilin University, Changchun, Jilin Province, People's Republic of China
[b] Department of Thoracic Surgery, First Teaching Hospital of Jilin University, Changhun, Jilin Province, People's Republic of China
[c] Department of Radiology, Institut Universitaire de Cardiologie et de Pneumologie de Québec, Canada
[d] Institut Universitaire de Cardiologie et de Pneumologie de Québec, Laval University, 2725 Chemin Sainte-Foy, Quebec City, Quebec G1V 4G5, Canada
* Corresponding author.
E-mail address: jean.deslauriers@chg.ulaval.ca

Thorac Surg Clin 21 (2011) 281–287
doi:10.1016/j.thorsurg.2010.12.009
1547-4127/11/$ – see front matter © 2011 Elsevier Inc. All rights reserved.

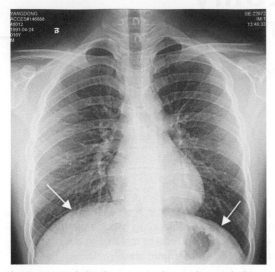

Fig. 1. Normal diaphragmatic domes (*arrows*) shown on a posteroanterior chest radiograph.

The muscular diaphragm can be depicted on cross-sectional studies such as CT or MR, although it is almost never seen in its full length because it is abutting neighboring structures of high densities such as the liver or spleen. On CT axial images, the anterior or sternocostal portion of the diaphragm is difficult to see unless it is delineated by peritoneal, retroperitoneal, or extraperitoneal fat (**Fig. 3**A) or fluid (see **Fig. 3**B). Posteriorly, the diaphragmatic crura that arise from the anterior aspects of the lumbar vertebral bodies can easily be seen on the direct CT axial planes (**Fig. 4**).

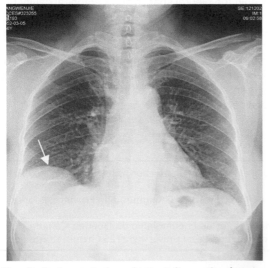

Fig. 2. Posteroanterior chest radiograph showing partial eventration of the right hemidiaphragm (*arrow*).

Three large openings disrupt the continuity of the diaphragm: the aortic hiatus, the esophageal hiatus, and the inferior vena cava hiatus. The aortic aperture, where transit the aorta, thoracic duct, and azygos vein, is the largest of these openings and is located behind the left median arcuate ligament at the level of T_{12}. Anterior to the aortic hiatus lies the esophageal hiatus through which run the esophagus, vagus nerves, and some esophageal arteries. It is located at the level of T_{10} and is best depicted on coronal and sagittal planes (**Figs. 5** and **6**). The esophageal hiatus is formed by the decussation of the medial fibers of the right crus, and its width increases with age, accounting for the higher prevalence of esophageal herniation in elderly people.[8,9] The most anterior and highest of the 3 diaphragmatic openings is the inferior vena cava hiatus, which transits the inferior vena cava and branches of the right phrenic nerve. It is located within the central tendon beneath the right atrium at the level of T_8-T_9.

ATTACHMENTS OF THE DIAPHRAGM

The sternocostal portion of the diaphragm is a muscular band that attaches to the xiphoid and lower 6 ribs (7 through 12). The most cephalic attachment is to the xiphoid (**Fig. 7**), giving it an inverted U-shaped configuration. On axial images, it can have 3 different types of configuration as reported by Gale.[8] In the most common configuration (type I) it has a relatively smooth soft-tissue curve, which is concave posteriorly and continuous with the lateral diaphragmatic arcs across the midline (**Fig. 8**). In type II configuration (**Fig. 9**), there is an anterior divergence and apparent discontinuity of muscle fibers as they insert onto the costal cartilages. On each image, the muscular line diverges rather than converges as it approaches the anterior chest wall. In type III configuration (**Fig. 10**), the middle leaflet is located inferior to the xiphoid. In the authors' experience, types II and III configurations are rarely seen on CT performed during shallow inspiration because in such cases, the middle leaflet of the central tendon is located cephalad to the xiphoid. By contrast, chest CT performed during deep inspiration shows a higher proportion of individuals with types II and III configurations because the middle leaflet of the central tendon is located more caudally during scanning time.

The posterior or lumbar portion of the diaphragm is made of 2 diaphragmatic crura, which are musculotendinous pillars arising from the upper 3 lumbar vertebrae. The 2 crura arch upward and forward to form the lateral margins of the aortic and esophageal hiatus. Both crura

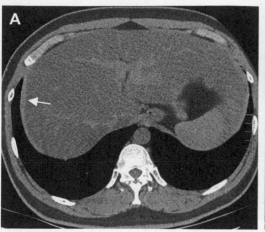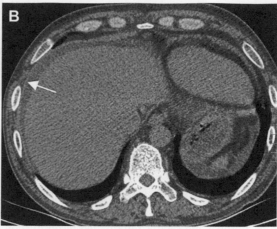

Fig. 3. (*A, B*) Delineation of the anterior diaphragm (*arrows*) in a patient with a fatty liver (*A*) and in another with peritoneal fluid (*B*).

connect in front of the aorta just above the celiac trunk through the fibrous medial arcuate ligament, which forms the anterior margin of the aortic hiatus.[1] Their size can be variable[10] and often they will appear lumpy or nodular on transaxial images. Maximal crural thickness ranges from 1.8 to 18.8 mm in men and from 1.8 to 21.1 mm in women, and this thickness does not change significantly during the various phases of the respiratory cycle. The crura form the anterior and lateral borders of the retrocrural spaces, and the presence of a strip of lung in this area may simulate free retroperitoneal air.

NORMAL DIAPHRAGMATIC ATTACHMENTS SIMULATING PATHOLOGIC PROCESSES

The normal diaphragmatic attachments and slips (folds of muscle protruding from the inferior surface of the diaphragm) can generate images

that simulate pathologic processes (**Fig. 11**). Diaphragmatic slips, for instance, are common, and they can show as wedge-shaped, round, oval, lobulated, or irregularly shaped structures.[10] With deep inspiration, the shortened and thickened diaphragmatic muscle fibers may indent the liver in a nodular or linear fashion.[3]

Occasionally the crura themselves may have a nodular appearance or an entire crus may simulate an enlarged lymph node on a single transaxial section, particularly on deep inspiration scans.[3,11] Misinterpretation of these images can be avoided by tracing these structures on contiguous sections.

A generalized increase in nodularity is often found in middle-aged and elderly individuals. Most commonly, these areas of nodularity lie over the mid-portion of the left hemidiaphragm, and they can be interpreted as localized enlargement or pseudotumors.[11]

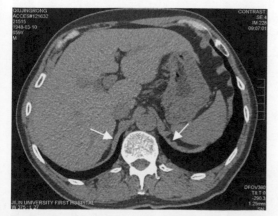

Fig. 4. CT scan showing the diaphragmatic crura (*arrows*).

DIAPHRAGMATIC DEFECTS AND AREAS OF WEAKNESSES

Asymptomatic posterolateral diaphragmatic defects found on CT in approximately 6% of normal individuals can mimic diaphragmatic tears. As described by Caskey and colleagues,[8] 3 types of defects in the diaphragmatic contours can be seen. Type I (**Fig. 12**) represents a localized defect in the thickness of the diaphragm, but the muscle continuity is maintained. In patients with type II abnormality (**Fig. 13**), there is an apparent defect in the diaphragm in which the muscle fibers appear to separate into layers parallel to the diaphragmatic contours, but the continuity of the diaphragm is maintained without protrusion of

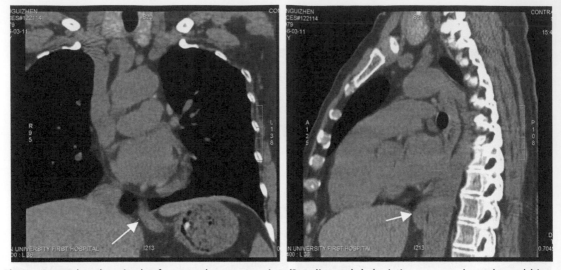

Fig. 5. Coronal and sagittal reformatted reconstruction (2 radiographs) depicting a normal esophageal hiatus and normal esophagus (*arrows*).

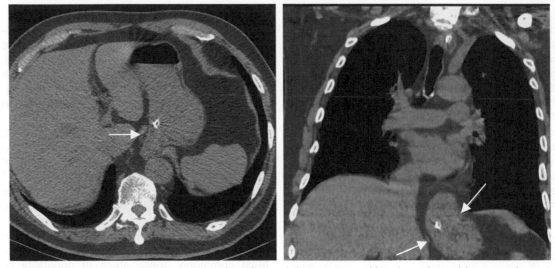

Fig. 6. CT scan with coronal reconstruction (2 radiographs) depicting a dilated esophageal hiatus with partial fundus herniation into the chest cavity (*arrows*).

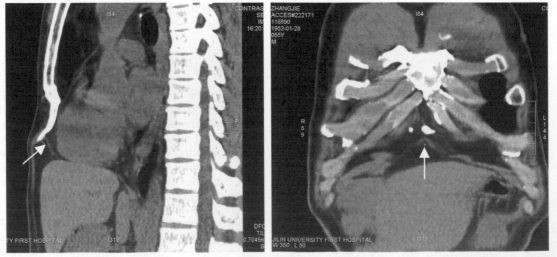

Fig. 7. Note the characteristic inverted U-shaped configuration (2 radiographs) of the anterior diaphragm with its apex at the level of the xiphoid (*arrows*).

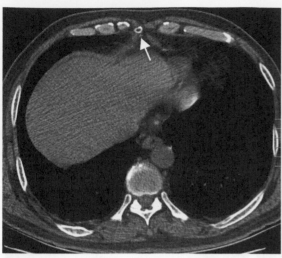
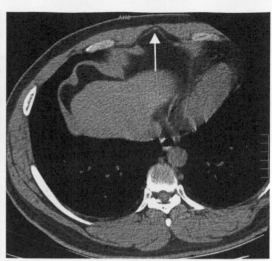

Fig. 8. Type I configuration (2 radiographs) of the anterior diaphragm where the middle leaflet of the central tendon is located cephalad to the level of the xiphoid and the liver is located behind the xiphoid (*arrows*). The anterior diaphragm shows as a thin curvilinear band that is concave posteriorly and continuous with the lateral fibers of the diaphragm across the midline.

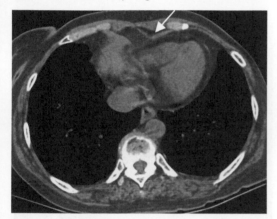

Fig. 9. Type II configuration of the anterior diaphragm where the middle leaflet of the central tendon is located caudal to the level of the xyphoid (*arrow*). The anterior diaphragmatic slips are orientated at an angle with the lateral fibers.

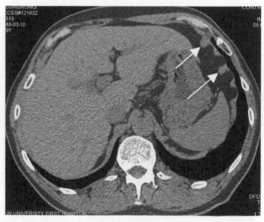

Fig. 11. Normal diaphragmatic slips simulating the presence of a mesothelioma (*arrows*).

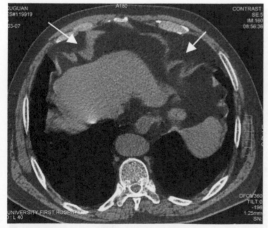

Fig. 10. Type III configuration of the anterior diaphragm where the middle leaflet of the central tendon is located at the same level as the xiphoid (*arrows*). The anterior diaphragm is a brood band with irregular and poorly defined margins.

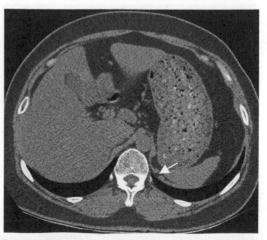

Fig. 12. Type I diaphragmatic defect. A low-attenuation area on the medial aspect of the posterior diaphragm gives rise to a localized defect (*arrow*) but the continuity of the muscle is maintained.

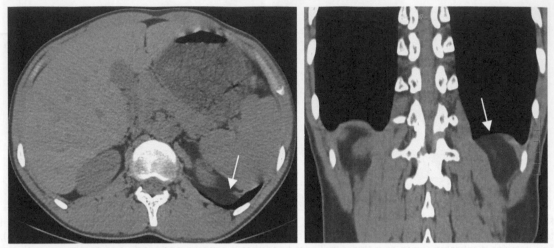

Fig. 13. Type II diaphragmatic defect (2 radiographs). Discontinuity of the posteromedial aspect of the diaphragm is shown on axial and coronal reformatted CT (*arrows*).

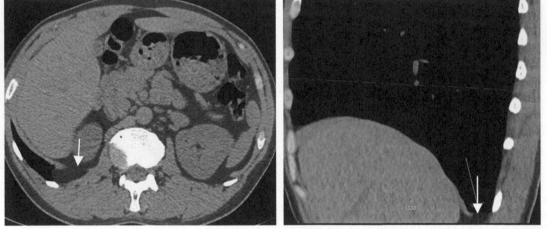

Fig. 14. Type III diaphragmatic defect (2 radiographs). Large defect in the left posterior diaphragm through which there is herniation of perirenal fat (*arrows*).

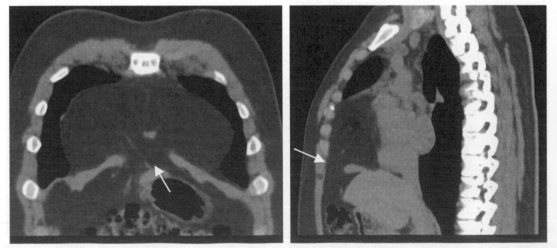

Fig. 15. Coronal and sagittal reformatted reconstruction depicting herniation (2 radiographs) of omental fat (Morgagni hernia) (*arrows*).

omental fat. Type III (**Figs. 14** and **15**) represents any defect in which a portion of the diaphragm is absent without loss of continuity. Protrusion of omental fat is a typical feature of these defects, which are seen predominantly on the left side and are thought to represent congenital asymptomatic Bochdalek hernias. As a rule, diaphragmatic defects are seen more commonly in women, in patients with emphysema, and in elderly individuals.

Partial eventration of the diaphragm (see **Fig. 2**) is thought to be a congenital disorder secondary to incomplete muscularization. It is composed of a thin membranous sheet replacing what would normally be muscle. Most eventrations involve the anteromedial portion of the right hemidiaphragm, and as the weakened area of muscle bulges cephalad, portions of the liver move upward.

SUMMARY

Imaging of the diaphragm is challenging because of its thin structure, complex shape, and close contact with the liver and spleen. Despite these difficulties, cross-sectional imaging studies, primarily CT and MRI, can depict normal anatomy as well as structural defects, both intrinsic and in adjacent organs. In this context, awareness of the anatomy of the diaphragm as well as of the correlation between anatomy and imaging is important if one wants to accurately diagnose diaphragmatic lesions.

REFERENCES

1. Panicek DM, Benson CB, Gottlieb RH, et al. The diaphragm: anatomic, pathologic, and radiologic considerations. Radiographics 1988;8:385–425.
2. Tarver RD, Conces DJ, Cory DA, et al. Imaging the diaphragm and its disorders. J Thorac Imaging 1989;4:1–18.
3. Gierada DS, Slone RM, Fleishman MJ. Imaging evaluation of the diaphragm. Chest Surg Clin N Am 1998;8:237–80.
4. Brink JA, Heiken JP, Semankovich J, et al. Abnormalities of the diaphragm and adjacent structures: findings on multiplanar spiral CT scans. AJR Am J Roentgenol 1994;163:307–10.
5. Naidich DP, Megibow AJ, Ross CR, et al. Computed tomography of the diaphragm: normal anatomy and variants. J Comput Assist Tomogr 1983;7:633–40.
6. Gierada DS, Curtin JJ, Erickson SJ, et al. Fast gradient echo magnetic resonance imaging of the normal diaphragm. J Thorac Imaging 1997;12:70–4.
7. Lennon EA, Simon G. The height of the diaphragm in the chest radiograph of normal adults. Br J Radiol 1965;38:937–43.
8. Caskey CI, Zerhouni EA, Fishman EK, et al. Aging of the diaphragm: a CT study. Radiology 1989;171:385–9.
9. Gale ME. Anterior diaphragm: variations in the CT appearance. Radiology 1986;161:635–9.
10. Callen PW, Filly RA, Koroskin M. Computed tomographic evaluation of the diaphragmatic crura. Radiology 1978;126:413–6.
11. Rosen A, Ho Auh Y, Rubenstein WA, et al. CT appearance of diaphragmatic pseudotumors. J Comput Assist Tomogr 1983;7:995–9.

General Anatomy of the Esophagus

Arzu Oezcelik, MD, Steven R. DeMeester, MD*

KEYWORDS
- Esophageal anatomy • Gastroesophageal junction
- Upper esophageal sphincter • Lower esophageal sphincter

EMBRYOLOGY OF THE ESOPHAGUS

The embryonic period extends from fertilization to the end of the eighth week and the fetal period starts at the ninth week and ends at birth. The digestive tube derives from 2 germ layers: the endoderm and the mesoderm. The endoderm is recognizable by the eighth day of the embryonic period. Until the third week, the embryo is a bilaminar disc of endoderm and ectoderm. Starting in the third week the mesoderm appears as a third embryonic layer, separating the endoderm and ectoderm. The mesoderm is the origin of the connective tissue, muscle coat, and serous coverings of the gut. The separation of the endoderm from the ectoderm allows the endoderm to undergo the extensive changes needed for the establishment of the embryonic primitive gut. The early digestive system forms during the fourth week and is divided into the foregut, the midgut, and the hindgut. The primitive foregut gives rise to the pharynx and its derivates, the esophagus, the trachea and lungs, the stomach and duodenum, the choledochal duct, the liver, the biliary system, and the pancreas.

GENERAL ANATOMY

The esophagus is a muscular tube that begins as the continuation of the pharynx in the neck and ends at the junction with the stomach. Normally, the transition from the pharynx to the esophagus occurs at the lower border of the sixth cervical vertebra. The esophagus descends anteriorly to the vertebral column through the middle mediastinum and traverses the diaphragmatic hiatus into the abdomen at the level of the tenth thoracic vertebral body (**Fig. 1**). After entering the abdomen it joins the stomach along the lesser curvature at what is called the cardia. The length of the entire esophagus ranges from 19 to 25 cm (median 22 cm) in men, and 18 to 22 cm (median 21 cm) in women.

The function of the esophagus is to transfer a bolus of material from the pharynx into the stomach. Deglutition is initiated when a bolus enters the pharynx from the oral cavity. Involuntary contraction of the pharyngeal muscles increases intrapharyngeal pressure and drives the bolus into the cervical esophagus. The upper esophageal sphincter relaxes precisely as intrapharyngeal pressure builds and allows the bolus to enter the esophagus. The contraction wave continues down the esophagus, pushing the bolus in an aboral direction. Distally, the lower esophageal sphincter (LES) relaxes on initiation of the swallow, and allows passage of the bolus into the stomach.

Topographically, the esophagus is divided into 3 regions: cervical, thoracic, and abdominal. The cervical esophagus is approximately 5 cm long and extends from the level of the sixth cervical vertebra to the level of the interspace between the first and second thoracic vertebrae posteriorly, and the suprasternal notch anteriorly. The cervical esophagus is bordered anteriorly by the trachea, posteriorly by the vertebral column and the prevertebral fascia, and laterally on each side by the carotid sheaths and the thyroid gland (**Fig. 2**). The buccopharyngeal fascia extends inferiorly on the posterior wall of the esophagus and laterally to the carotid sheaths and separates the esophagus from the prevertebral fascia. These fascial

Department of Surgery, Keck School of Medicine, University of Southern California, 1510 San Pablo Street, Los Angeles, CA 90033, USA
* Corresponding author.
E-mail address: sdemeester@surgery.usc.edu

Thorac Surg Clin 21 (2011) 289–297
doi:10.1016/j.thorsurg.2011.01.003

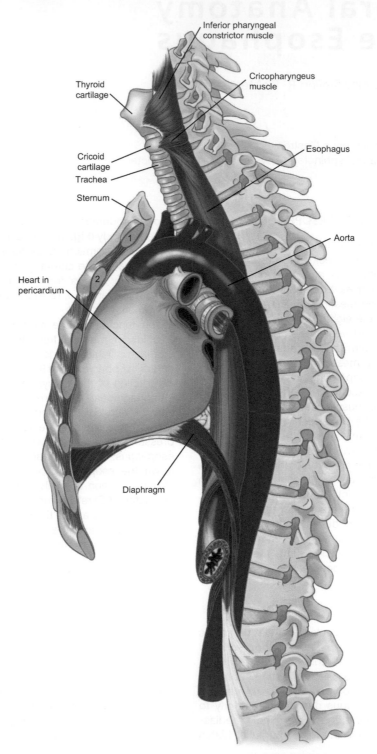

Fig. 1. The esophagus descends anteriorly to the vertebral column through the middle mediastinum and traverses the diaphragmatic hiatus into the abdomen at the level of the tenth thoracic vertebral body.

planes form a paraesophageal space and a retroesophageal and create compartments that allow extension of cervical infections into the mediastinum.

The thoracic esophagus is approximately 20 cm long and extends from the thoracic inlet to the diaphragmatic hiatus. From the thoracic inlet to the tracheal bifurcation the thoracic esophagus is

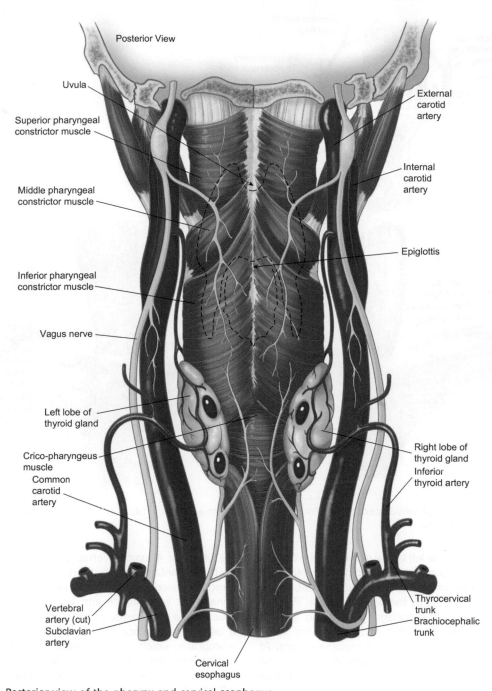

Posterior View

Uvula

Superior pharyngeal
constrictor muscle

Middle pharyngeal
constrictor muscle

Inferior pharyngeal
constrictor muscle

Vagus nerve

Left lobe of
thyroid gland

Crico-pharyngeus
muscle
Common
carotid
artery

Vertebral
artery (cut)
Subclavian
artery

External
carotid
artery

Internal
carotid
artery

Epiglottis

Right lobe of
thyroid gland
Inferior
thyroid artery

Thyrocervical
trunk
Brachiocephalic
trunk

Cervical
esophagus

Fig. 2. Posterior view of the pharynx and cervical esophagus.

related anteriorly to the membranous wall of the trachea and posteriorly to the prevertebral fascia and spine. The esophagus descends posterior to the aortic arch and then lies to the right of the descending thoracic aorta, and posterior and to the right of the subcarinal lymph nodes and the pericardium (**Fig. 3**). At the level of the eighth thoracic vertebra the esophagus moves anterior to the aorta and then enters the esophageal hiatus at the level of the tenth thoracic vertebra. The right lateral surface of the thoracic esophagus is covered by parietal pleura. The left lateral surface of the thoracic esophagus is covered proximally by the left subclavian artery and the parietal

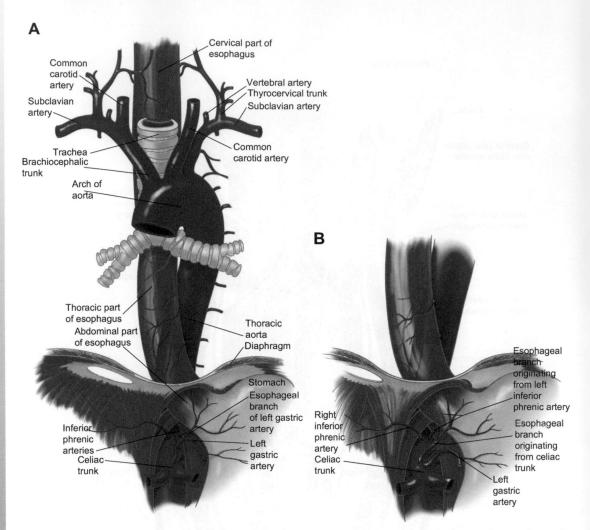

Fig. 3. (*A*) The esophagus descends posterior to the trachea adn aortic arch. (*B*) At the hiatus the esophagus lies anterior to the aorta.

pleura. Distally the left lateral surface of the esophagus is covered by the descending thoracic aorta until the level of the eighth thoracic vertebra and subsequently only by the parietal pleura. Posteriorly, the thoracic esophagus remains in contact with the vertebral bodies and follows the spine until the level of the eighth thoracic vertebra. At this level the esophagus moves anterior to the aorta and enters through the esophageal hiatus into the abdomen.

The abdominal portion of the esophagus begins once the esophagus transits the diaphragmatic hiatus and ends when it joins the cardia of the stomach along the high lesser curvature. The intra-abdominal length of the esophagus is typically 2 to 6 cm long. The right and left crura of the diaphragm form the esophageal hiatus and are composed of muscular fibers that arise as tendinous bands from the anterolateral surface of

the first 3 or 4 lumbar vertebrae. The abdominal aorta lies anterior to the vertebral bodies, and directly posterior to the esophageal hiatus. The vena cava lies inferior and lateral to the right crus. As the esophagus passes through the hiatus it becomes enveloped in the phrenoesophageal membrane, which is a fibroelastic sheet of tissue arising from the subdiaphragmatic fascia. Within the abdomen, the esophagus lies posterior to the left lateral segment of the liver.

GASTROESOPHAGEAL JUNCTION

The gastroesophageal junction is the location where the esophagus joins the stomach (**Fig. 4**). Although seemingly straightforward, controversy continues today about the precise location of the gastroesophageal junction. The difficulty is in part related to the method used to identify the gastroesophageal

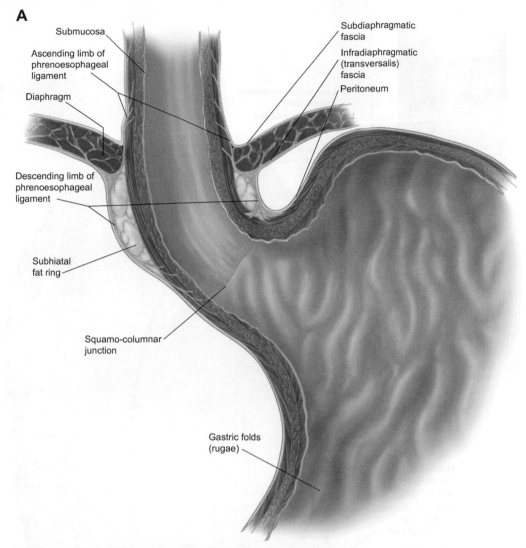

Fig. 4. (*A*) The precise location of the gastroesophageal junction remains controversial based to some extent how it is determined. (*B*) The muscle layers of the esophagus and stomach.

junction: endoscopic, surgical, histologic, or pathologic. Some of the definitions include:

- The location of the peritoneal reflection onto the stomach
- The location of the junction between the tubular esophagus and the saccular stomach
- The region adjacent to the acute angle of His
- The distal extent of the white esophageal squamous epithelium
- The proximal extent of gastric oxyntic mucosa
- The proximal limit of the gastric rugal folds
- The manometric distal end of the LES
- The point beyond which no submucosal esophageal glands are found

- The change in the muscularis propria from a circular and longitudinal layer in the esophagus to a less defined muscularis propria of the stomach with a third oblique layer.

Although these criteria have all have been used to define the gastroesophageal junction, some are pathologic or histologic criteria, some endoscopic, and some surgical, and because all 3 approaches are rarely available at once, the correlation between them remains ambiguous. With damage to the distal esophagus from gastroesophageal reflux and development of a hiatal hernia, the landmarks and relationships of structures around the gastroesophageal junction become altered, and the identification of the precise gastroesophageal junction becomes more complicated.

B

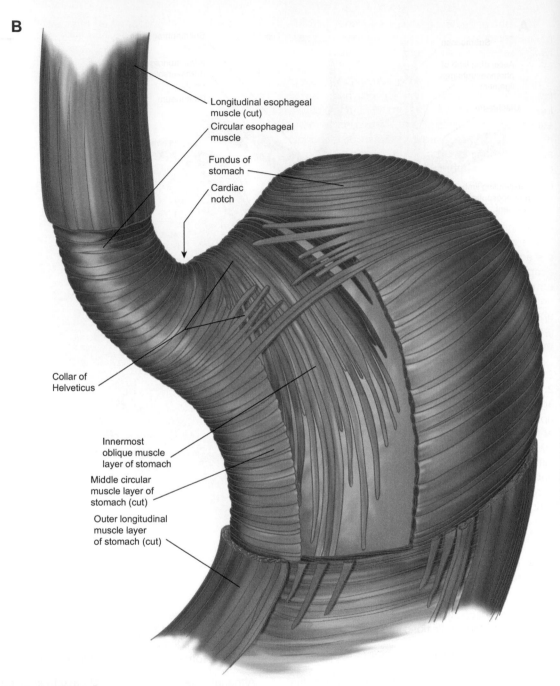

Longitudinal esophageal muscle (cut)

Circular esophageal muscle

Fundus of stomach

Cardiac notch

Collar of Helveticus

Innermost oblique muscle layer of stomach

Middle circular muscle layer of stomach (cut)

Outer longitudinal muscle layer of stomach (cut)

Fig. 4. (*continued*)

HISTOLOGY

The wall of the esophagus consists of 4 layers: mucosa, submucosa, muscularis propria, and adventitia. Unlike other areas of the gastrointestinal tract it does not have a serosal layer.

The mucosa consists of 3 layers:

- Epithelium: squamous epithelium, bordered inferiorly by the basement membrane

- Lamina propria: thin layer of connective tissue below the basement membrane above the muscularis mucosa
- Muscularis mucosa: a thin layer of longitudinally and irregularly arranged smooth muscle fibers that separate the mucosa from the submucosa. It is thin in the proximal part of the esophagus and becomes thicker distally.

The submucosa separates the mucosa and the muscularis propria. It contains blood vessels, lymph vessels, nerves, and elastic and collagen fibers.

The muscularis propria consists of an internal layer of circular fibers and an external layer of longitudinal fibers. In the proximal third of the esophagus the muscularis propria is striated muscle. At approximately the level of the aortic arch it transitions into smooth muscle, and in the distal two-thirds of the esophagus the muscularis propria consists only of smooth muscle. Between the external longitudinal muscle layer and the internal circular muscle layer is a neuronal network called the myenteric plexus.

The outermost layer of the esophageal wall is the adventitia. It is a fibrous layer that covers the esophagus, connecting it with neighboring structures. It is composed of loose connective tissue and contains small vessels, lymphatic channels, and nerve fibers. Unlike the other portions of the gastrointestinal tract, the esophagus is not lined by serosa.

The dimensions of the upper esophagus are 2.5 cm by 1.6 cm and the lower esophagus 2.5 cm by 2.4 cm. There are 3 areas in the esophagus where the lumen normally narrows. The uppermost normal anatomic narrowing is located at the entrance into the esophagus and is caused by the cricopharyngeus muscle. The average luminal diameter at this point is 1.5 cm and is the narrowest point of the esophagus. The second narrowing is in the area where the left mainstem bronchus and the aortic arch cross the esophagus. The average luminal diameter at this point is 1.6 cm. The lowermost narrowing is at the hiatus, where the esophagus leaves the chest and enters the abdomen. The luminal diameter at this point is 1.6 cm. These 3 areas of anatomic narrowing are of importance in that swallowed foreign objects tend to hold up at 1 of these locations.

The esophagus has 2 intrinsic high-pressure zones called the upper esophageal sphincter and the LES. These regions of high pressure are similar to the other areas of the esophagus, and are not identifiable on gross or microscopic examination of the esophagus. Instead, these areas are only identifiable using manometry and measuring the pressure within the lumen of the esophagus.

THE UPPER ESOPHAGEAL SPHINCTER

The upper esophageal sphincter (UES) is a high-pressure zone separating the pharynx from the esophagus. The length varies between 2 and 4 cm. It prevents entry of air into the digestive tract during inspiration and reflux of esophageal contents into the hypopharynx after swallowing. During a swallow it relaxes and opens to allow the bolus to enter the cervical esophagus.

The UES is a musculocartilaginous structure composed of the cricoid cartilage, the hyoid bone and 3 muscles: cricopharyngeus, cervical esophagus, and inferior pharyngeal constrictor (**Fig. 5**). The cricopharyngeus is the most definitive component of the UES. It is composed of striated muscle fibers that are attached to the cricoid cartilage. It forms a C-shaped muscular band with

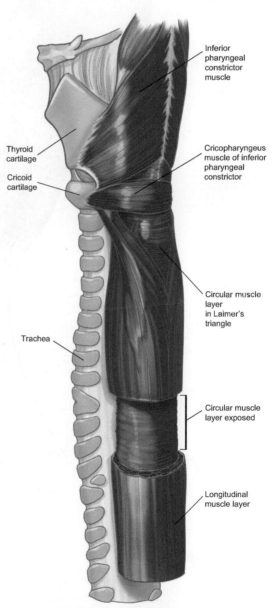

Fig. 5. The UES is a musculocartilaginous structure composed of the cricoid cartilage, the hyoid bone, and 3 muscles: cricopharyngeus, cervical esophagus, and inferior pharyngeal constrictor.

maximum tension in the anteroposterior rather than lateral direction. It is composed of a mixture of fast- and slow-twitch muscle fibers, with the slow fibers being predominant. This mixture enables the cricopharyngeus to maintain constant basal tone yet have a rapid response during swallowing, belching, and vomiting. The cervical esophagus is similar to the cricopharyngeus in that it contains predominantly slow fibers. The muscle fibers are arranged in an external longitudinal layer, and an internal circular layer. The inferior pharyngeal constrictor is the thickest of the 3 muscles and contains 2 layers: a thick external layer of predominantly fast-twitch fibers and

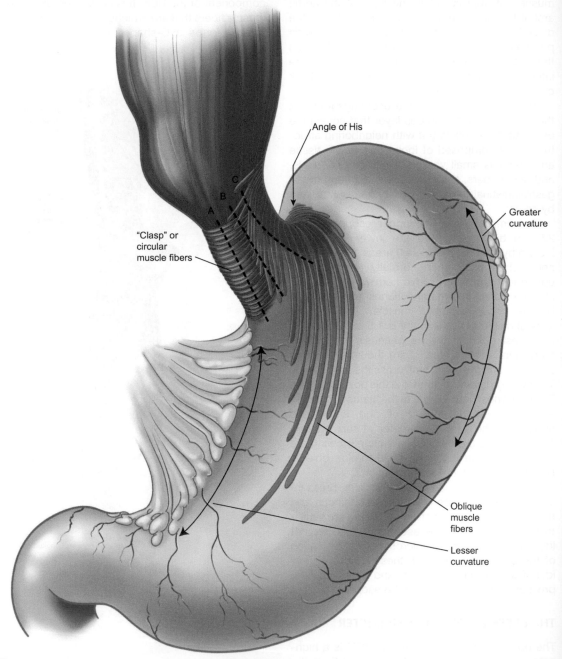

Fig. 6. The LES splays out onto the cardia of the stomach as clasp fibers, which are short semi-circular muscle fibers along the lesser curvature, and sling fibers, which are short and long oblique muscular fibers along the greater curvature and angle of His. The ideal location for a Heller myotomy in patients with achalasia is unknown, but results may differ based on which fibers are disrupted, as illustrated by the lines A, B and C.

a thin inner layer of predominantly slow-twitch fibers. Given the structural similarity of the inner layer of the inferior pharyngeal constrictor to the cricopharyngeus, it is likely that the inner layer of the inferior pharyngeal constrictor functions similar to the cricopharyngeus.

THE LES

The LES is a high-pressure zone in the distal esophagus near the gastroesophageal junction. It is the main barrier against reflux of gastric juice into the esophagus. The sphincter is a physiologic region of increased or basal pressure, but there are no grossly or microscopically identifiable features or specific morphologic changes in the musculature at the site of the LES. Identification of the LES can only be done with a manometry study. Using manometry, the LES is 2 to 4 cm long with a resting pressure of 15 to 20 mm Hg. Three-dimensional manometric assessment of the LES has shown marked radial and longitudinal asymmetry, with the highest pressure in the left posterior direction.

Normally the LES spans the hiatus, and therefore has both a thoracic and abdominal component. The thoracic part of the LES is 1 to 2 cm long and the abdominal portion is another 1 to 2 cm long, for a total length of a normal LES of 2 to 4 cm. The total length, abdominal length, and resting pressure of the LES function together to create resistance to retrograde flow of gastric contents into the negative pressure environment of the thoracic esophagus. The LES splays out onto the cardia of the stomach as clasp fibers, which are short semi-circular muscle fibers along the lesser curvature, and sling fibers, which are short and long oblique muscular fibers along the greater curvature and angle of His (**Fig. 6**). These terminal muscle fibers may have particular relevance for the location of a myotomy in patients with achalasia.

SUMMARY

The esophagus is a muscular tube approximately 22 cm in length that functions to transport a bolus from the mouth to the stomach. It begins as the continuation of the pharynx in the neck and ends at the gastroesophageal junction. Topographically, it is divided into cervical, thoracic, and abdominal components, and each area has unique features and associations with surrounding structures. On histology, the esophageal wall consists of 4 layers: mucosa, submucosa, muscularis propria, and adventitia. The esophagus has 2 intrinsic high-pressure zones called the UES and the LES, which prevent reflux from the esophagus into the hypopharynx and from the stomach into the esophagus.

FURTHER READINGS

Blevins CE. Embryology of the esophagus. In: Shields TW, LoCicero J, Ponn RB, et al, editors. General thoracic surgery. International Textbook of Medicine, vol. 2. 6th edition. Philadelphia: Lippincott Williams & Wilkins; 2005. p. 1881–4.

Duranceau A, Liebermann-Meffert D. Embryology, anatomy, and physiology of the esophagus. In: Zuidema GD, editor. Shackelford's surgery of the alimentary tract. International Textbook of Medicine, vol. 1. 3rd edition. Philadelphia: WB Saunders; 2002. p. 3–39.

Hagen JA, DeMeester TR. Anatomy of the esophagus. In: Shields TW, LoCicero J, Ponn RB, et al, editors. General thoracic surgery. International Textbook of Medicine, vol. 2. 6th edition. Philadelphia: Lippincott Williams & Wilkins; 2005. p. 1885–93.

Lang IM, Shaker R. An overview of the upper esophageal sphincter. Curr Gastroenterol Rep 2000;2(3): 185–90.

Liebermann-Meffert D. Clinically oriented anatomy, embrology, and histology. In: Patterson GA, Cooper JD, Deslauriers J, et al, editors. Pearson's thoracic & esophageal surgery. International Textbook of Medicine, vol. 2. 3rd edition. Philadelphia: Churchill Livingstone Elsevier; 2008. p. 10–28.

Singh S, Hamdy S. The upper oesophageal sphincter. Neurogastroenterol Motil 2005;17(Suppl 1):3–12.

Sivarao DV, Goyal RK. Functional anatomy and physiology of the upper esophageal sphincter. Am J Med 2000;108(Suppl 4a):27S–37S.

The Esophageal Wall

Thomas W. Rice, MD[a,b,*], Mary P. Bronner, MD[a,c]

KEYWORDS

- Mucosa • Submucosa • Muscularis propria
- Adventitia • Lymphatics

The sole function of the esophagus is transport of solid and liquid nourishment from the pharynx to the stomach and, rarely, venting of the stomach with retrograde passage of gastric contents into the pharynx. What appears to be a simple task is provided by a complex and not completely understood organ. To investigate, diagnose, and treat both benign and malignant esophageal diseases, an in-depth understanding of the esophageal wall is required.

THE ESOPHAGEAL WALL

The esophageal wall is a four-layer structure with a mucosa, submucosa, muscularis propria, and adventitia (**Fig. 1**).

Mucosa

The mucosa is composed of the epithelium and its basement membrane, the lamina propria, and the muscularis mucosae.

Epithelium and basement membrane

The esophagus is lined by stratified nonkeratinizing squamous epithelium (**Fig. 2**). Unlike the skin, it is a moist surface and lacks appendages other than the ducts of submucosal glands. Its role is to protect the underlying esophageal wall from mechanical damage, microorganisms, and toxic materials. However, it is not keratinizing as in mammals that eat coarse food. The esophageal epithelium is continuous with pharyngeal epithelium. It ends abruptly at the squamocolumnar junction, which resides in the distal 2 to 3 cm of the tubular esophagus in normal individuals, a region also known as the lower esophageal sphincter. The normal squamocolumnar mucosal junction does not necessarily align with the gastroesophageal junction, the anatomic junction of the tubular esophagus, and the saccular stomach. The gastroesophageal junction is the site at which the proximal-most radiating gastric folds terminate. Thus, the normal squamocolumnar mucosal junction can be located anywhere from the gastroesophageal anatomic junction to 2 to 3 cm above it. The mucosa distal to the squamocolumnar junction, also known as the z-line, is gastric cardiac and fundic glandular epithelium (**Fig. 3**).

The epithelium has three layers: basal cell, prickle cell, and functional cell. The basal cell layer (stratum basale or stratum germinativum) is 1 to 3 cells thick and is the source of epithelial regeneration. It occupies 10% to 15% of the epithelium, except in the distal esophagus, where a thickness of more than 15% may still be normal. Progressive maturation with flattening of cells occurs within the epithelium as it extends onto the epithelial surface. The boundary between the basal cell and prickle cell layers is arbitrarily defined as the point at which nuclei are separated by a distance no greater than their diameter. The prickle cell (stratum spinosum) is so named because of the shrinkage artifact that exposes the adhesion between cells at their desmosomal junctions. The cells in the functional layer maintain their nuclei, and although they do not keratinize, they may

Supported in part by the Daniel and Karen Lee Endowed Chair in Thoracic Surgery.
[a] Cleveland Clinic Lerner College of Medicine of Case Western Reserve University, East 100 Street, Cleveland, OH 44106, USA
[b] Cleveland Clinic, Department of Thoracic and Cardiovascular Surgery, 9500 Euclid Avenue/Desk J4-1, Cleveland, OH 44195, USA
[c] GI Pathology, Molecular Morphologic Pathology, Department of Anatomic Pathology, Cleveland Clinic, Cleveland, OH 44195, USA
* Corresponding author. Cleveland Clinic Lerner College of Medicine of Case Western Reserve University, Cleveland, OH.
E-mail address: ricet@ccf.org

Thorac Surg Clin 21 (2011) 299–305
doi:10.1016/j.thorsurg.2011.01.005

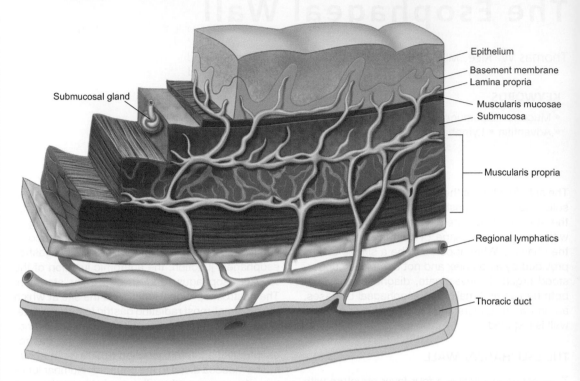

Epithelium
Basement membrane
Lamina propria
Muscularis mucosae
Submucosa
Submucosal gland
Muscularis propria
Regional lymphatics
Thoracic duct

Fig. 1. The esophageal wall is a four-layer structure, with a mucosa, submucosa, muscularis propria, and adventitia. The mucosa is a three-layer structure, with an epithelium and its basement membrane, lamina propria, and muscularis mucosae. (*Adapted from* Cleveland Clinic Foundation, 1999; with permission.)

occasionally demonstrate keratohyalin granules. In humans, esophageal epithelium turnover is approximately 21 days.[1]

Lymphocytes are normally found above the basal cell layer. The conformational changes necessary for their intracellular position between progressively flattening epithelial cells give them

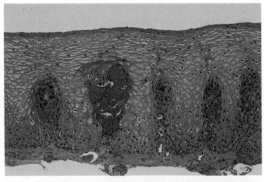

Fig. 2. Stratified nonkeratinizing squamous epithelium of normal esophageal mucosa, demonstrating the 1- to 2-cell-thick basal layer occupying no more than 15% of the mucosal thickness and the gradual flattening of the squamous cells as the epithelium matures to the mucosal surface. Note also that the subepithelial papillae of lamina propria extend no higher than two-thirds of the epithelial thickness (hematoxylin and eosin).

an appearance termed a "squiggle cell." This can mimic the segmented nucleus of a granulocyte, except that lymphocytic squiggle cells lack the cytoplasmic granules of either a neutrophil or an eosinophil. Argyrophil-positive endocrine cells[2] and rare melanocytes[3] are also found in normal basal cell layers and are the cells of origin for neuroendocrine carcinomas, including small-cell carcinoma, of the esophagus and primary esophageal melanoma, respectively.

The findings of squamous hyperplasia, regeneration, and intraepithelial inflammation (**Fig. 4**) are nonspecific signs of esophagitis most typically, but not necessarily, resulting from gastroesophageal reflux disease. Epithelial hyperplasia is defined by basal cell hyperplasia (more than 15% of the mucosal thickness occupied by basal cells) or papillomatosis (elongation of the subepithelial papillae of lamina propria to more than two-thirds of the mucosal thickness). Intraepithelial inflammatory cells comprise neutrophils, eosinophils, and lymphocytes.

Glandular epithelium in the tubular esophagus may derive from congenital ectopic columnar epithelium (inlet-patch within the proximal esophagus) or an acquired columnar lining (Barrett esophagus), a metaplastic response to chronic gastroduodenal reflux into the distal esophagus.

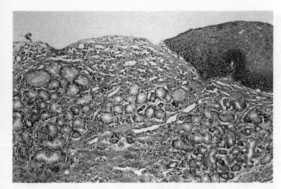

Fig. 3. The squamocolumnar junction, z-line, stratified nonkeratinizing squamous epithelium on the right and gastric cardia mucosa on the left (hematoxylin and eosin).

Specialized columnar epithelium, characterized by the presence of intestinal metaplasia with goblet cells, is required for the diagnosis of Barrett esophagus, regardless of the site of biopsy within the esophagus. This epithelium is characterized by two principal cell types: goblet cells and nongoblet columnar cells. Goblet cells are barrel-shaped and have a distended, mucin-filled cytoplasm (**Fig. 5**). Histochemically, goblet cells contain acid mucins that stain positively with Alcian blue at pH 2.5. The columnar cells in between goblet cells may resemble either gastric foveolar cells (typical of incomplete intestinal metaplasia) or intestinal pseudoabsorptive cells (typical of complete intestinal metaplasia). Unlike normal gastric foveolar cells, which contain neutral mucin, nongoblet columnar cells in either reflux disease or Barrett esophagus may contain Alcian blue at pH 2.5-positive

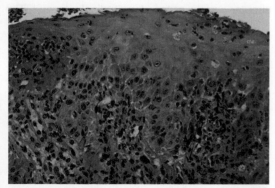

Fig. 4. Squamous hyperplasia, regeneration, and intraepithelial inflammation of esophagitis, the most common cause of which is gastroesophageal reflux disease, as in this case. Note the expansion of the basal cell layer of the squamous mucosa as a feature of hyperplasia, the nuclear enlargement of the squamous cells as a feature of regeneration, and the intraepithelial neutrophils and eosinophils that are also important elements of the diagnosis of esophagitis (hematoxylin and eosin).

acid mucin. These cells have been called "tall columnar blues." In the absence of goblet cells, a diagnosis of Barrett esophagus should not be rendered based solely on the presence of columnar blues.

The basement membrane anchors the epithelium to the lamina propria and isolates the epithelium from the remainder of the esophageal wall. It is composed of type IV collagen. Destruction of the basement membrane by malignant cells originating in the epithelium is the first step of cancer invasion and thus defines an invasive carcinoma, distinguishing it from high-grade dysplasia (in situ carcinoma). The basement membrane is also the antigenic stimulus for autoimmune esophageal dermatologic diseases, such as pemphigus, pemphigoid, and epidermolysis bullosa.

Lamina propria

The lamina propria (lamina propria mucosae) is a thin layer of loose connective tissue containing a complex of collagen and elastic fibers. It contains a network of endothelial-lined channels, both capillaries and lymphatics, that provide intramucosal carcinoma with access to hematogenous or lymphatic spread. This is the main reason that carcinoma with the potential for metastasis is first seen at the intramucosal level within the esophagus, and it is why pathologists must carefully examine this compartment in esophageal neoplasia. Scattered inflammatory cells, including lymphocytes and plasma cells, are normally found in the lamina propria.

Muscularis mucosae

The muscularis mucosae is composed of a longitudinal layer of smooth muscle and exhibits regional differences.[4] In the cervical esophagus, it is sparse with scattered muscle bundles within a matrix of connective tissue. In the thoracic esophagus, it is well developed and consists of several bundles. In the distal esophagus, it has a reticular pattern with bundles running in various directions. The esophageal muscularis mucosae is the thickest muscularis mucosae of the entire gastrointestinal tract and can even approach the thickness of the muscularis propria. Knowledge of this is important in assessing the greatest depth of invasive carcinoma within the esophageal wall, particularly on endoscopic mucosal resections or even esophagectomy specimens. The robust thickness of the esophageal muscularis mucosae can easily be mistaken for the muscularis propria. Whereas blood vessels and glandular ducts pierce the muscularis mucosae nearly vertically in areas of underdevelopment, lymphatic vessels take a more oblique or longitudinal path.[4]

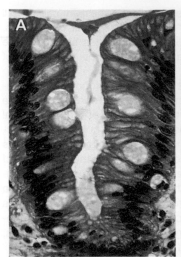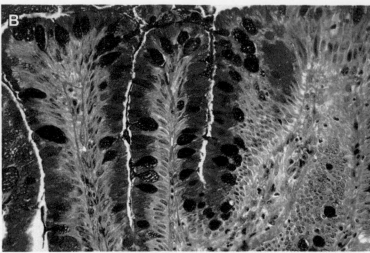

Fig. 5. Barrett esophagus (*A*) Specialized columnar epithelium with goblet cells, also known as intestinal meta-plasia, which is an essential and defining element of Barrett esophagus. Note that there are actually multiple cell types in this epithelium, including not only the defining and barrel-shaped goblet cell, but also the inter-vening nongoblet columnar cells that resemble mixtures of both gastric surface foveolar-type cells and intestinal absorptive-type cells with poorly formed luminal brush borders (pseudoabsorptive cells; hematoxylin and eosin). (*B*) Goblet cells contain acid mucins that stain positively with Alcian blue at pH 2.5.

The role of the muscularis mucosae in swallow-ing is not completely understood, but it is believed to both permit and limit dilatation during passage of the food bolus, providing a buffer against the increased pressure gradient between the esopha-geal lumen and thoracic cavity. However, the mucosal contribution to the strength of the esoph-agus is not developed until the outer esophageal diameter is doubled.[5] Absence of the muscularis mucosae has been reported in patients with poste-metic esophageal rupture (Boerhaave syndrome).[6] Duplication of the muscularis mucosae in patients with columnar-lined esophagus is common, but its development and significance relative to cancer staging in particular are not understood.[7] The nature of lymphatic passage through and arrange-ment around the muscularis mucosae has been speculated to be a reason for the low prevalence of regional lymph node metastases in mucosal (superficial) cancers of the esophagus.[4]

Submucosa

The submucosa is composed of loose connective tissue containing blood vessels, lymphatics, nerves, and submucosal glands. These glands are similar to minor salivary glands in the pharynx and are present in the esophagus but not the stomach (**Fig. 6**). They produce acid mucin, bicar-bonate, water, electrolytes, epidermal growth factor, and prostaglandins, providing a variety of epithelial protective functions.[8] The ducts arising from the glands pass through the mucosa to

discharge into the esophageal lumen. The cuboidal lining cells of these ducts may be a source of repair for the esophageal mucosa, but are not a path for cancer invasion.[9] Rare primary esophageal adeno-carcinomas may derive from the submucosal glands or ducts, and these conform to the same subtypes occurring in oropharyngeal salivary gland tumors.

Muscularis Propria

The muscularis propria is composed of an inner circular and outer longitudinal layer. The

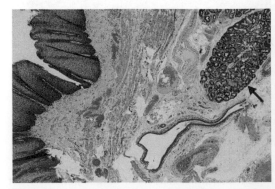

Fig. 6. Submucosal gland (*arrow*) and an accompa-nying duct. The glands have a lobulated or rounded clustering of simple mucinous glands. These submu-cosal glands are not present in the stomach and are a histologic landmark for defining anatomic esoph-agus. The dark blue coloration of the mucinous cyto-plasm reveals that they secrete acid mucin on this special stain (Alcian blue at pH 2.5).

circular layer is a complex helical structure, responsible for peristalsis. The proximal 4% to 5% of the esophagus is composed completely of striated muscle and the distal 54% to 62% of smooth muscle.[10] The transition from striated to smooth muscle in the circular muscle layer is gradual, and the 50-50 point is approximately 5 cm from the cricopharyngeus muscle. This transition is always more distal in the longitudinal muscle layer. Unlike the upper esophageal sphincter, which is distinct, the lower esophageal sphincter is not a readily identifiable structure. The circular muscle of the distal 2 to 6 cm of the esophagus thickens to approximately twice that of the immediately adjacent muscularis mucosae.[11]

Adventitia

The esophagus lies in a bed of fat, neurovascular and connective tissue and elastic fibers termed the adventitia. Unlike the stomach, small bowel, and colon, it has no serosa, except in its short abdominal segment.

ARTERIAL SUPPLY

The blood supply of the esophagus derives from multiple small segmental vessels. These are typically less than 1 mm in diameter and pass for a number of centimeters from their origin before branching at or in the esophageal wall. The cervical esophagus is supplied by branches from the superior and inferior thyroid arteries and on occasion by direct branches of the subclavian artery. The thoracic esophagus receives its blood supply from tracheal and bronchial arteries. Although up to two esophageal branches arising directly from the aorta have been reported, no esophageal branches have been found in a third of autopsies.[12] Intercostal arteries by themselves, and sometimes through bronchial and tracheal arterial branches, may also supply the thoracic esophagus. The abdominal esophagus receives its blood supply, along with the proximal stomach, from the left gastric and splenic arteries.

When these arteries reach the esophagus, their orientation is horizontal to the axis of the esophagus in the upper esophagus and vertical in the lower.[12] In thoracic esophagus, these arteries branch in the periesophageal tissue before entering the esophageal wall. Elegant corrosion casts of the esophageal blood supply demonstrate the dense vascular network within the mucosa and submucosa, which is the terminus of these arteries.[12]

This unique esophageal blood supply allows extensive esophageal mobilization and esophageal devascularization for varices without necrosis and transhiatal (blunt) esophagectomy without exsanguination.

VENOUS DRAINAGE

Effluent from the scanty capillary network of the lamina propria drains into a coarse polygonal meshwork of veins in this layer.[13] In turn, this plexus drains into veins that perforate the muscularis mucosae. On entering the submucosa, these veins turn horizontally and unite to form 10 to 15 longitudinal veins that form a submucosal plexus midway between the muscularis mucosae and muscularis propria.[13] In the proximal esophagus, this plexus has fewer veins of larger diameter; whereas, in the distal esophagus, there are more submucosal veins of smaller diameter. In the distal esophagus, these two plexi communicate directly with their counterparts in the stomach and permit decompression of the portal venous system in portal hypertension.[14,15]

The submucosal plexus drains by perforating veins, which acquire tributaries as they pass through the muscularis propria. Valves directing venous flow out of the esophagus are first seen in these veins.[13] The point of exit is usually on the right-posterior and left-anterior borders of the esophagus in close association with the vagus nerves. These veins drain into regional large veins. In the neck, drainage is via the inferior thyroid and brachiocephalic veins, in the thorax, via the azygos and hemiazygos veins and their tributaries, and in the abdomen, via the left gastric and splenic veins.

LYMPHATIC DRAINAGE

The delicate and collapsed nature of lymphatics precludes study by injection techniques used to produce casts of the vascular esophageal anatomy. Lymphatic vessels are identifiable in the mucosa and submucosa on routine histologic preparation of the esophageal wall. These findings, plus the relationship between lymph node metastases and cancer invasion, led to speculation on the existence of a rich network of lymphatics in the mucosa and submucosa mirroring the arterial and venous anatomy.[16] However, recent immunohistochemical study of the esophageal wall using lymphatic endothelial marker D2–40 has provided new insight into the lymphatic anatomy of the esophageal wall.[17] There is a dense longitudinal plexus of lymphatic vessels in the lamina propria. Rare perforating lymphatics have been found draining into a sparse circumferential lymphatic network in the outer margin of the submucosa. Perforating lymphatics from the submucosal plexus, usually running with an artery and vein, penetrate the inner circular layer of the muscularis propria. Here, they drain into a circumferential intramuscular plexus that accompanies the artery, vein, and nerves of this space. Afferent lymphatics, usually accompanied by an artery and vein, drain the intramuscular plexus into the lymphatic channels in the adventitia. No direct connection from the lamina propria network and the thoracic duct was identified.[17]

There are marked differences in the adventitial lymphatic system according to the side of the esophagus on which the lymphatic is found.[18] Lymphatic drainage from the right side of the esophagus is longitudinal and multistationed. However, longitudinal lymphatics are poorly developed on the left side of the esophagus, and frequent drainage is seen into the thoracic duct.[18] Existence of direct routes from mural lymphatics to the thoracic duct, without a relay through regional lymphatics and lymph nodes, has been documented by many investigators. However, the exact patterns and occurrence of these pathways are highly variable.[18–21] Although regional lymph nodes are found along the course of the extramural lymphatic network, they are generally concentrated. The major hub occurs at the tracheobronchial bifurcation and pulmonary hilum. These nodes drain both the esophagus and lung, and the direction of lymph flow may be either cephalad or caudad. Below this, most lymph flow generally proceeds caudad. At the distal esophagus, another concentration of regional lymph nodes, albeit a more diffuse distribution, occurs and includes lymph nodes at the esophagogastric junction, cardia, and omentum. Above the tracheal bifurcation, lymph typically flows cephalad to neck nodes in the region of the trachea and tracheoesophageal groove.

NERVE SUPPLY

The esophagus has dual innervation from the vagus (parasympathetic) and spinal afferent nerves (sympathetic). These systems exert antagonistic effects on muscle, glands, and blood vessels. The parasympathetic nervous system provides motor innervation to the esophageal musculature and sphincters, producing peristalsis and sphincter relaxation. It supplies secretomotor innervation to esophageal glands. The sympathetic nervous system exerts the opposite effect on the esophageal musculature and glands and produces vasoconstriction. These nerves pass with blood vessels and lymphatics into the esophageal wall. There is a neural network in the esophageal wall composed of fine nerve fibers and numerous ganglia. The networks lie between the two muscle layers of the muscularis propria (Auerbach plexus) and in the submucosa (Meissner plexus).

SUMMARY

The esophagus spans three body cavities and has no mesentery, continually borrowing or sharing vessels, lymphatics, and nerves with associated organs. However, constant along this path is an intricate mural structure. An understanding of the esophageal wall, its blood supply, lymphatic drainage, and innervation is essential for successful esophageal surgery.

REFERENCES

1. Squier CA, Kremer MJ. Biology of oral mucosa and esophagus. J Natl Cancer Inst Monogr 2001;29:7–15.
2. Tateishi R, Taniguchi K, Horai T, et al. Argyrophil cell carcinoma (apudoma) of the esophagus. A histopathologic entity. Virchows Arch A Pathol Anat Histol 1976;371(4):283–94.
3. DiCostanzo DP, Urmacher C. Primary malignant melanoma of the esophagus. Am J Surg Pathol 1987;11(1):46–52.
4. Nagai K, Noguchi T, Hashimoto T, et al. The organization of the lamina muscularis mucosae in the human esophagus. Arch Histol Cytol 2003;66(3):281–8.
5. Goyal RK, Biancani P, Phillips A, et al. Mechanical properties of the esophageal wall. J Clin Invest 1971;50(7):1456–65.
6. Kuwano H, Matsumata T, Adachi E, et al. Lack of muscularis mucosa and the occurrence of Boerhaave's syndrome. Am J Surg 1989;158(5):420–2.
7. Abraham SC, Krasinskas AM, Correa AM, et al. Duplication of the muscularis mucosae in Barrett esophagus: an underrecognized feature and its implication for staging of adenocarcinoma. Am J Surg Pathol 2007;31(11):1719–25.
8. Long JD, Orlando RC. Esophageal submucosal glands: structure and function. Am J Gastroenterol 1999;94(10):2818–24.
9. Tajima Y, Nakanishi Y, Tachimori Y, et al. Significance of involvement by squamous cell carcinoma of the ducts of esophageal submucosal glands. Analysis of 201 surgically resected superficial squamous cell carcinomas. Cancer 2000;89(2):248–54.
10. Meyer GW, Austin RM, Brady CE 3rd, et al. Muscle anatomy of the human esophagus. J Clin Gastroenterol 1986;8(2):131–4.
11. Apaydin N, Uz A, Elhan A, et al. Does an anatomical sphincter exist in the distal esophagus? Surg Radiol Anat 2008;30(1):11–6.

12. Liebermann-Meffert DM, Luescher U, Neff U, et al. Esophagectomy without thoracotomy: is there a risk of intramediastinal bleeding? A study on blood supply of the esophagus. Ann Surg 1987;206(2):184–92.

13. Butler H. The veins of the oesophagus. Thorax 1951; 6(3):276–96.

14. Kitano S, Terblanche J, Kahn D, et al. Venous anatomy of the lower oesophagus in portal hypertension: practical implications. Br J Surg 1986; 73(7):525–31.

15. Vianna A, Hayes PC, Moscoso G, et al. Normal venous circulation of the gastroesophageal junction. A route to understanding varices. Gastroenterology 1987;93(4):876–89.

16. Rice TW, Zuccaro G Jr, Adelstein DJ, et al. Esophageal carcinoma: depth of tumor invasion is predictive of regional lymph node status. Ann Thorac Surg 1998;65(3):787–92.

17. Yajin S, Murakami G, Takeuchi H, et al. The normal configuration and interindividual differences in intramural lymphatic vessels of the esophagus. J Thorac Cardiovasc Surg 2009;137:1406–14.

18. Saito H, Sato T, Miyazaki M. Extramural lymphatic drainage from the thoracic esophagus based on minute cadaveric dissections: fundamentals for the sentinel node navigation surgery for the thoracic esophageal cancers. Surg Radiol Anat 2007;29(7):531–42.

19. Riquet M, Le Pimpec Barthes F, Souilamas R, et al. Thoracic duct tributaries from intrathoracic organs. Ann Thorac Surg 2002;73(3):892–8 [discussion: 898–9].

20. Kuge K, Murakami G, Mizobuchi S, et al. Submucosal territory of the direct lymphatic drainage system to the thoracic duct in the human esophagus. J Thorac Cardiovasc Surg 2003;125(6): 1343–9.

21. Murakami G, Sato I, Shimada K, et al. Direct lymphatic drainage from the esophagus into the thoracic duct. Surg Radiol Anat 1994;16(4):399–407.

Correlative Anatomy for the Esophagus

Paula A. Ugalde, MD[a],*, Sergio Tadeu Pereira, MD[a],
Cesar Araujo, MD[b]

KEYWORDS

- Esophagus • Anatomy • Diagnostic imaging

The esophagus is a muscular tube connecting the pharynx to the stomach, acting as a channel for the transport of food. A comprehensive knowledge of the anatomy is essential to understand esophageal disease states.

Imaging of the hollow organs of the gastrointestinal tract began more than a century ago. By the beginning of the twentieth century, barium sulfate suspensions had emerged as the contrast agent of choice for opacification and radiographic examination of the gastrointestinal tract. By the 1970s, fiber-optic endoscopy and computed tomography (CT) had been invented and developed into complementary ways of imaging the digestive system.

Because the esophagus is a tubular muscular structure only partially filled with air and surrounded by major structures[1] (vessels, lungs and heart), its radiologic evaluation cannot be performed solely by conventional chest radiograph (**Fig. 1**) or barium studies. Knowledge of the surfaces contacted by the esophagus throughout its extension from the neck to the abdomen allows an understanding of the anatomic relationships with all neighboring structures.

The emergence of newer techniques has had a dramatic effect on the use of luminal contrast examinations of the gastrointestinal tract. This article describes the current radiographic techniques for examining the gastrointestinal tract with contrast materials, emphasizing the role of barium suspensions, CT scan, and magnetic resonance imaging (MRI), and illustrating normal anatomy.

OVERVIEW OF THE ESOPHAGEAL ANATOMY

The esophagus commences at the pharyngoesophageal junction at the lower border of the sixth cervical vertebra. It is formed primarily by the cricopharyngeus muscle[2] and ends at the cardia at the level of the eleventh thoracic vertebra.[3] It is approximately 25 to 30 cm long, most of this being in the thorax, with short cervical and intraabdominal segments (**Figs. 2** and **3**).[4] It is a muscular tube lined by stratified squamous epithelium with outer longitudinal and inner circular muscle fibers.[5] The internal circumference has 2 to 3 cm in the relaxed state.[6] In adults, in general, at 40 cm from the incisors the gastroesophageal junction can be identified.[4] The cardia normally has a high resting tone or pressure,[3] which begins to relax approximately 3 seconds after the swallowing wave starts, thus allowing the food bolus to enter the stomach.[5,7]

The esophagus has several important relationships in its course through the thorax (see **Figs. 2** and **3**). The cervical part is related anterior to the trachea, common carotid artery, and thyroid gland (**Fig. 4**). The thoracic part begins in the anterosuperior mediastinum (**Fig. 5**) and then progresses toward the posterior mediastinum. It passes to the right of the aortic arch and then descends next to the descending aorta on the

Funding: none.
[a] Department of Thoracic Surgery, Santa Casa de Misericordia Hospital, Praça Cons Almeida Couto #500, Centro Medico Celso Figueroa, Sala 207, Nazaré 40000, Salvador-Ba, Brazil
[b] Radiology Department, Federal University of Bahia School of Medicine, Salvador, Bahia, Brazil
* Corresponding author.
E-mail address: paugalde@terra.com.br

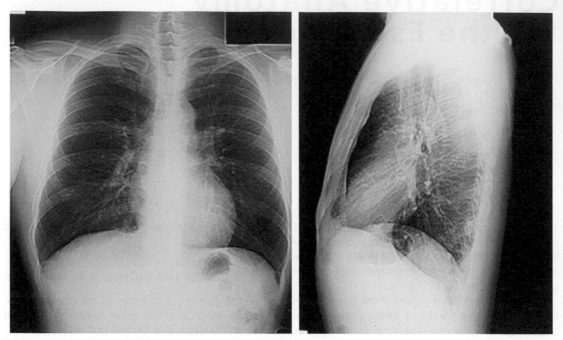

Fig. 1. Frontal and lateral chest radiograph without oral contrast; this is not an ideal examination to evaluate the esophagus because it cannot be outlined.

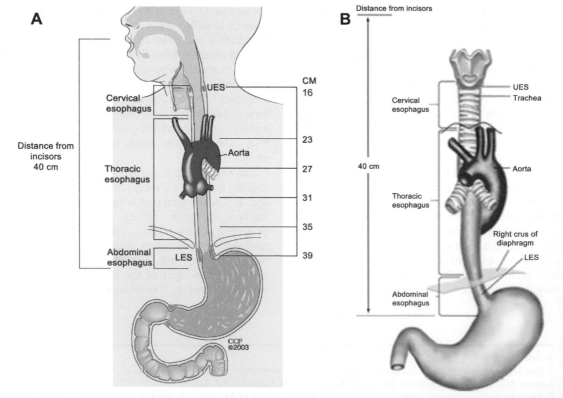

Fig. 2. Diagram of the esophagus and major neighboring structures. The esophagus is approximately 20 to 25 cm long, originates in the neck at the level of the cricoid cartilage, passes through the chest, and ends after passage through the hiatus by joining the stomach below (*A, B*). ([A] Reprinted with permission, Cleveland Clinic Center for Medical Art & Photography © 2003–2011. All Rights Reserved.)

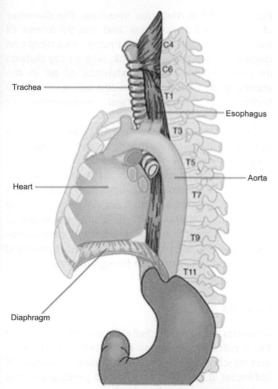

Fig. 3. Diagram of a lateral view of the esophagus and its correlation with the spine, airway, mediastinum, and abdominal contents.

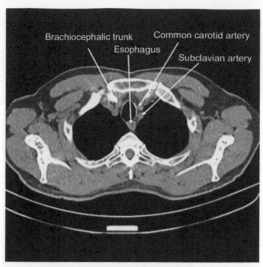

Fig. 5. Chest CT scan. At the thoracic inlet the trachea is anterior but shifts slightly to the right of the esophagus, and the lungs are posterior and lateral. The left subclavian, common carotid arteries, the brachiocephalic artery, and the brachiocephalic veins can be identified at this level.

the left lobe of the liver, finishing at the gastroesophageal (GE) junction (**Fig. 7**).[5,8]

PLAIN RADIOGRAPHY

In general, plain radiographs without oral contrast add little useful information to the esophageal

left side. Its main anterior relationships are the left main bronchus, the pericardium, and the heart. Along the right side, the esophagus is bordered by the pleura and the azygos vein (**Fig. 6**). A short segment passes through the diaphragm next to

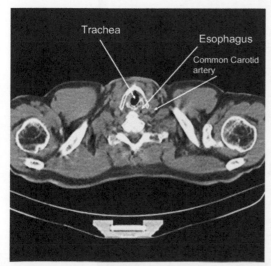

Fig. 4. Chest CT scan at the cervical portion of the esophagus and its correlation with the trachea and common carotid artery.

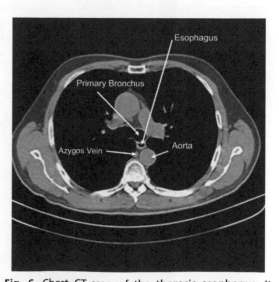

Fig. 6. Chest CT scan of the thoracic esophagus. It passes between the aorta and the azygos vein toward the abdomen. Anteriorly are the left main bronchus, the pericardium, and the heart. Note that the esophagus is bordered by the mediastinal pleura along its length.

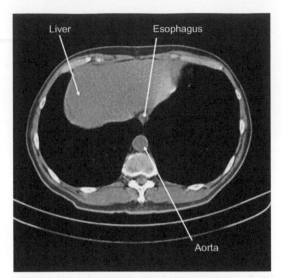

Fig. 7. Chest CT scan of the distal esophagus at the level of the thoracoabdominal transition. Note the proximity to the left lobe of the liver and the distance to the aorta at this level.

evaluation because this is a midline flat structure (see **Fig. 1**). Its appearance in the resting state is determined by the neighboring structures and the pressure within the cavities it traverses.

Because of the muscular structure, the diameter of the normal esophagus and the thickness of the esophageal wall in image examinations depend on the presence of air, which may distend its internal lumen.[9] The existence of air in the esophageal lumen is considered an unusual finding on routine chest radiograph or esophagography.[9]

Occasionally, in patients who have a dilated gas-filled esophagus, the right esophageal wall may be shown on chest radiographs, marked by the esophagopleural stripe and the azygoesophageal line.[9] If present, these lines may be distorted in certain conditions, such as carcinoma of the esophagus. Otherwise, there is no routine use of plain radiography in the assessment of esophageal disease, with the exceptions of suspected perforation or radiopaque foreign bodies.

BARIUM STUDIES

A barium study is the ideal examination to evaluate the swallowing, passage of the bolus, peristalsis, and function of the upper and lower esophageal sphincter (LES) and to rule out perforation and endoluminal obstruction.[4]

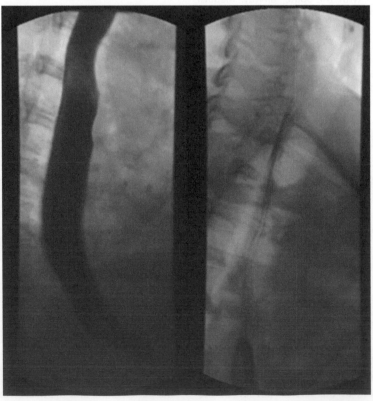

Fig. 8. Barium esophagogram. Fluoroscopic examination of the esophagus. Note the passage of the oral contrast in a fully distended and coated esophagus.

The examination starts with the patient erect and turned obliquely to the left, so that the body of the esophagus is thrown clear of the spine. A barium suspension at 100% weight/volume is standard, because this allows good mucosal coating and yet is not too dense. With the patient horizontal and in the right anterior oblique position the barium study allows the evaluation of motility of the esophagus and full distention of the GE junction can be accomplished. The fully distended and coated esophagus has a smooth mucosal surface, as seen both in profile and en face (**Fig. 8**).[5]

The initial bolus is observed fluoroscopically as a fast shot to ascertain if there is any obvious structural abnormality. Although essentially a midline structure, the esophagus deviates slightly to the left in the neck and to the right in the thorax, following the curvature of the vertebral column. Then it curves to the left again as it passes through the hiatus in the diaphragm at the level of T10 (**Fig. 9**).[10,11]

The cervical portion of the esophagus is flattened because of compression of adjacent structures, the thoracic portion is more rounded because of the negative intrathoracic pressure, and the abdominal portion is flat again because of the positive intraabdominal pressure. Also, there are 3 normal areas of anatomic narrowing

in the esophagus[5]: at the entrance of the esophagus caused by the cricopharyngeus muscle, at the level of the crossing of the left main stem bronchus and the aortic arch, and at the hiatus because of the pressure of the LES (**Fig. 10**).[7] These areas of normal constriction are important because swallowed foreign objects tend to hold up at these points.

In cases in which esophageal rupture or tear is suspected, opacification with water-soluble contrast agent is imperative. If an ionic contrast agent such as Gastrografin (meglumine diatrizoate) is aspirated, it can cause severe pulmonary problems. In practice, a nonionic water-soluble contrast agent such as Gastromiro (iopamidol) is the best option. If this agent fails to show any obvious leak, it may be followed by a barium esophagogram.

The passage of the bolus is marked by the primary peristalsis, which is a muscular contraction that propels the bolus downward and collapses the lumen of the esophagus.[7] Any residual barium is then cleared by a secondary wave initiated by esophageal distention or gastric reflux rather than by swallowing. Tertiary waves are sometimes seen, particularly in elderly patients, and these usually consist of nonpropulsive disorganized contractions that fail to advance the barium bolus.[12]

The swallowing mechanism is then checked at the pharyngoesophageal phase.[2] This inspection allows the pick-up of functional disorders of the hypopharynx or the upper esophageal sphincter, Zenker diverticulum, and extrinsic compression caused by low thyroid goiter. At the level of the

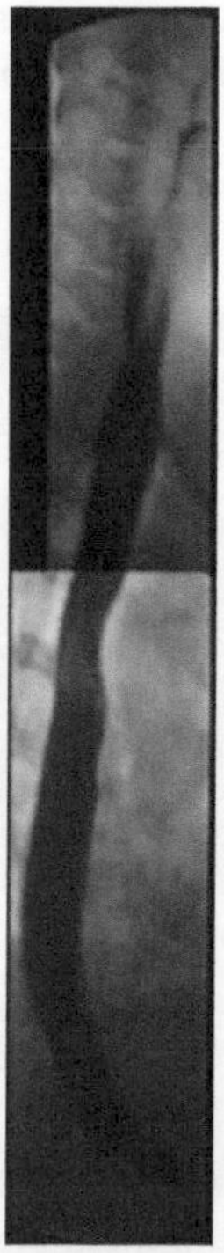

Fig. 9. Barium esophagogram. Lateral view of the esophageal course from the crycopharingeous muscle to the GE junction.

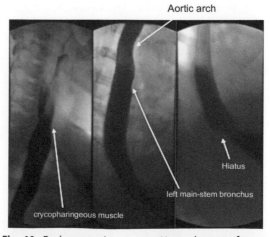

Aortic arch

crycopharingeous muscle

left main-stem bronchus

Hiatus

Fig. 10. Barium esophagogram. Normal areas of anatomic narrowing in the esophagus: at the entrance of the esophagus, at the level of the crossing of the left main stem bronchus and the aortic arch, and at the hiatus.

thoracic esophagus, the swallow study may reveal achalasia, diffuse esophageal spasm, esophageal diverticula, benign or malignant tumors, compression by aberrant vascular anomalies, or compression by mediastinal posterior tumors or by an enlarged left atrium. At the GE junction (**Fig. 11**) the deglutition of barium allows verification of normal pliability of the lower esophagus, function of the LES, congenital short esophagus, hiatus hernia, mucosal appearance, and esophageal varices.[7]

For patients complaining of "food sticking in the back of the throat," choking, or concerned about aspiration pneumonia, a modified barium swallow is the preferred technique. However, in cases of dysphagia, odynophagia, or heartburn, a barium esophagogram should be the first choice. Full-distention views with continuous swallowing assess morphology to rule out tumor, stricture, ulcer, and so forth. Fold thickening is a frequent but nonspecific manifestation of esophagitis either secondary to infection or to reflux. Mucosal erosion and ulceration are characteristic of reflux esophagitis, which can be recognized as streaks or dots of barium against the flat mucosa of the esophagus.[11]

CT

The hallmark of normal CT anatomy of the esophagus is the delineation of mediastinal tissue planes throughout its extent. Therefore, knowledge of the normal relationship between the esophagus and other mediastinal structures allows the recognition of pathologic alterations produced by esophageal disease.[13]

The neck, thorax, and upper abdomen should always be examined. The administration of intravenous contrast is essential to highlight the vessels, and the use of oral contrast helps distend the stomach and opacify the entire length of the esophagus during scans acquisition.[13] In the chest, the superior and inferior boundaries are at the level of the T4 vertebral body and the diaphragm, respectively. The thoracic esophagus, the descending aorta, and the azygos vein should be clearly delineated as separate and distinct structures on every slice in a normal patient (**Fig. 12**).

Although the esophagus is easily recognized on thoracic CT, little attention has been directed toward its normal and abnormal appearance. CT plays no substantial role in the evaluation of most benign esophageal diseases.[14]

The role of a CT scan in the assessment of esophageal disease is mainly:

1. To evaluate and stage patients with esophageal carcinoma and to provide means for assessing response to therapy and resultant complications
2. To evaluate and characterize esophageal contour abnormalities detected at the esophagography and their relationship to intrinsic or extrinsic masses
3. To evaluate patients with suspected esophageal perforation and to assess the extent of pleural and mediastinal involvement.

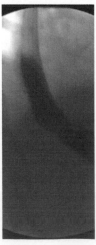

Fig. 11. Barium esophagogram. Detail of the GE junction after oral contrast.

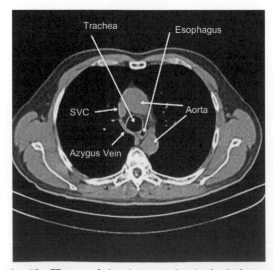

Fig. 12. CT scan of the chest. Mediastinal window at the level of the distal trachea. Note the correlation of the esophagus with the aorta, azygos, trachea, and superior vena cava.

The development of positron emission tomography CT has added a major new role for CT scan in the assessment of esophageal malignancy, because the involvement of nodes or liver can now be more accurately assessed.

Cervical Esophagus

The cervical esophagus is a relatively midline structure posterior to the trachea (**Fig. 13**). In the neck, lack of sufficient paraesophageal fat makes differentiation of the esophagus from adjacent soft tissues more difficult. Furthermore, density artifacts from the adjacent cervical vertebrae and bones of the shoulder girdle detract from the image. As a result, unless oral contrast is present CT of the cervical esophagus is not warranted because of these difficulties.[14]

Thoracic Esophagus

The relation of the thoracic esophagus to the other mediastinal structures should be described on a regional basis.[14]

From the thoracic inlet to the tracheal bifurcation, the thoracic esophagus is intimately related to the posterior wall of the trachea and the prevertebral fascia. At the thoracic inlet the trachea remains anterior but shifts slightly to the right of the esophagus, and the lungs are posterior and lateral. Vascular structures that may be appreciated at this level include the left subclavian and common carotid arteries laterally on the left, the brachiocephalic artery anterolaterally on the right, and the brachiocephalic veins further laterally (**Fig. 14**).

At the level of the aortic arch, the esophagus remains a relatively midline structure. Anterior and to the right is the trachea, laterally on the right are the lymph nodes and superior vena cava, and to the left is the ascending aorta (**Fig. 15**). The thoracic spine is posterior. The retrotracheal space should not exceed 4 mm, or a pathologic process should be suspected.

At the level of the tracheal bifurcation, the airway has moved toward a midline position, immediately anterior to the esophagus. The descending aorta lies posterolateral to the esophagus on the left side, and on the right side is the azygos vein (**Fig. 16**). The lungs are immediately beside the esophagus at this level.

Just caudal to the carina, the esophagus is in intimate contact with the left main stem bronchus (**Fig. 17**). This relationship accounts for the frequent occurrence of esophagobronchial fistula in advanced esophageal carcinoma. However, these 2 structures are clearly separable from one another. Below this level, the esophagus maintains a fairly constant proximity to the posterior wall of the left atrium, a relation that accounts for the external compression of the esophageal wall in patients with left atrium enlargement. From there down, the esophagus passes over the posterior surface of the subcarinal lymph nodes, and then descends behind the pericardium to reach the diaphragmatic hiatus. It lies just to the left of the midline and anterior to the descending aorta (**Fig. 18**).

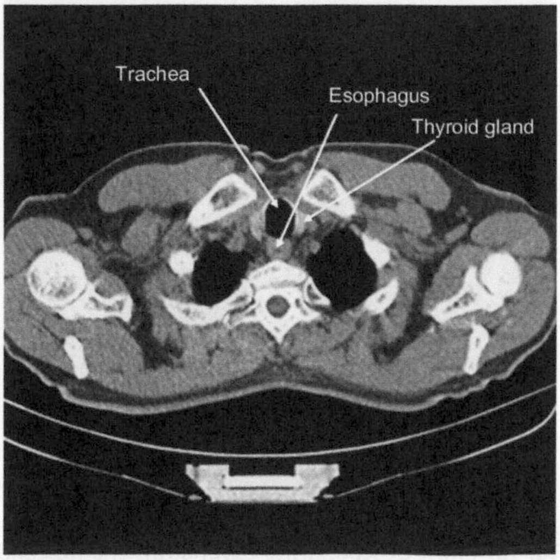

Fig. 13. Chest CT scan. The cervical esophagus as a midline structure posterior to the trachea and lateral to the thyroid gland.

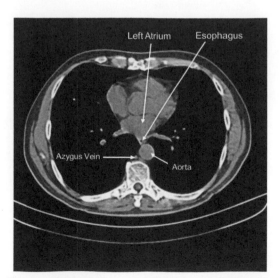

Fig. 14. Chest CT scan. The thoracic esophagus, the descending aorta, and the azygos vein are clearly delineated as separate and distinct structures on every slice.

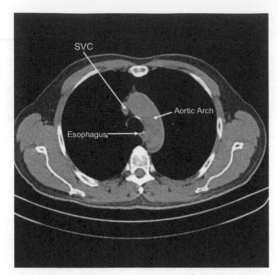

Fig. 15. Chest CT scan at the level of the aortic arch. Anterior and to the right is the trachea, on the right side are the lymph nodes and superior vena cava, and to the left is the ascending aorta. The thoracic spine is posterior.

The descending aorta, azygos vein, and inferior vena cava maintain the same interaction to the esophagus as they pass through the diaphragm. However, as the esophagus traverses the diaphragmatic hiatus it begins a leftward migration before entering the cardia of the stomach.[15] As the esophagus passes through the hiatus it is surrounded by the phrenoesopageal membrane, which ultimately merges as the visceral peritoneal coverage of the stomach.[10,12]

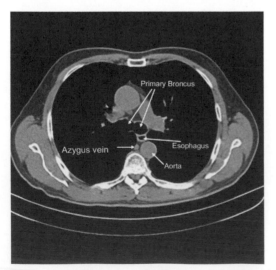

Fig. 16. Chest CT scan at the level of the tracheal bifurcation. The descending aorta lies on the left side of the esophagus, and on the right side is the azygos vein.

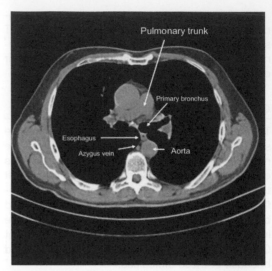

Fig. 17. Chest CT scan caudal to the carina. The esophagus is in intimate contact with the left main stem bronchus.

Air is commonly detected radiographically in the normal esophagus, but how much, how often, and in what distribution is not well known.[6,9] Air in the esophagus above the azygos and aortic arches outlines the inner right and left esophageal walls (Fig. 19). The right and left lungs delineate the outer esophageal walls as they approach each other. At the level of the aortic and azygos branches, esophageal air again outlines the inner wall of the esophagus. The outer wall is not outlined because the aortic and azygos arches prevent the lung from contacting the left and right

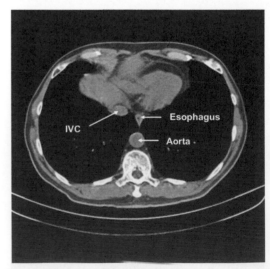

Fig. 18. Chest CT scan: distal esophagus. The descending aorta, azygos vein, and inferior vena cava maintain the same interaction to the esophagus as they pass through the diaphragm.

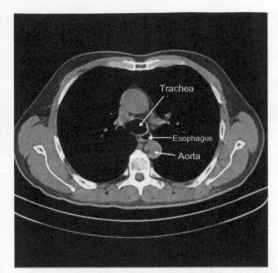

Fig. 19. Chest CT scan. Air in the esophagus outlines the inner right and left esophageal walls.

For recommendations of normality, we can say that air is normal in the esophagus, but distention of more than 10 mm at a prespecified fixed point, such as the carina, is uncommon.[6] Also, the normal LES should be closed, with no air inside.

MRI

There are no definite protocols for esophageal MRI, but there are some basic necessities. Cardiac gating may be needed to reduce the problem of motion artifact. Both T1- and T2-weighted imaging is necessary, ideally using breath-hold (eg, gradient echo) sequences. Images in coronal and sagittal planes may be helpful in addition to the standard axial sequences (**Figs. 20** and **21**).

esophageal walls, respectively. However, esophageal air below the azygos and aortic arches again draws the inner esophageal walls until the proximity with the LES.[9]

Advances in MRI technology have enabled development of high-spatial-resolution imaging sequences (small field of view, thin slices). Recognition of specific resection planes with MRI allows preoperative means of predicting resectability of esophageal tumors and thus aids in selection of patients for surgery.[16] However, to our knowledge high-resolution MRI has not been developed for imaging the esophagus.

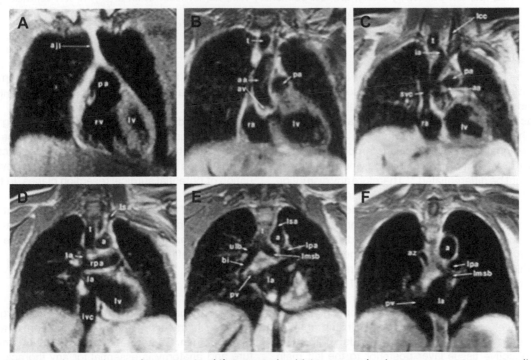

Fig. 20. Normal coronal scans from anterior (*A*) to posterior (*F*) in a normal volunteer. a, aorta; an, ascending aorta; ajl, anterior junction line; av, aortic valve; az, azygos vein; bi, bronchus intermedius; ia, innominate artery; ivc, inferior vena cava; la, left atrium; lbcv, left brachiocephalic vein; lcc, left common carotid artery; lmsb, left main stem bronchus; lpa, left pulmonary artery; lsa, left subclavian artery; lv, left ventricle; pa, main pulmonary artery; pv, pulmonary vein; ra, right atrium; rpa, right pulmonary artery; rv, right ventricle; svc, superior vena cava; t, trachea; ta, truncus anterior; ulb, upper lobe bronchus.

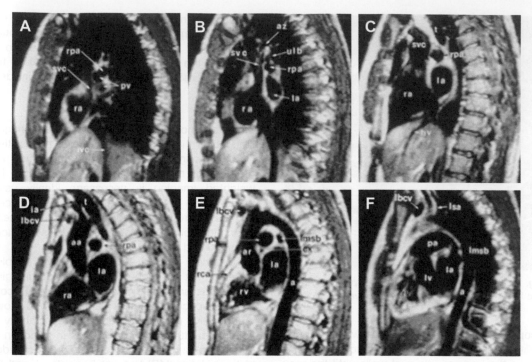

Fig. 21. Contiguous sagittal scans of hila and mediastinum from left (*A*) to right (*F*) in a normal volunteer. a, aorta; aa, ascending aorta; ar, aortic root; az, azygos vein; cx, circumflex coronary artery; hv, hepatic vein; ia, innominate artery; ivc, inferior vena cava; la, left atrium; lbcv, left brachiocephalic vein; lmsb, left main stem bronchus; lpa, left pulmonary artery; lpv, left pulmonary vein; lsa, left subclavian artery; lv, left ventricle; pa, main pulmonary artery; pv, pulmonary vein; ra, right atrium; rca, right coronary artery; rpa, right pulmonary artery; rv, right ventricle; svc, superior vena cava; t, trachea; ulb, upper lobe bronchus.

The layers of the esophageal wall can be clearly visible on high-resolution MRI.[16] Normal mucosa produced a fine intermediate signal layer, which was often corrugated. This layer was surrounded by high-signal-intensity submucosa and the outer low-signal-intensity muscularis propria. However, with T1-weighted imaging the individual wall layers cannot be differentiated.[17] Therefore any disruption of the layers of the gastrointestinal tract, by tumor for example, is likely to be better delineated with the fast spin-echo T2-weighted technique.[16,18]

Recent MR images identified a distinct fascial layer that passes posterior to the esophagus within the posterior mediastinum and condenses bilaterally with the parietal pleura. This layer may provide the lateral and posterior margins for surgical resection of the lower esophagus up to the level of the pulmonary veins. In the anterior aspect, periesophageal fat extends to the thin connective tissue layer posterior to the left main bronchus and inferior in relation to the fibrous pericardium. The MR images highlighted the intimate relation between the esophagus and the posterior wall of the left main bronchus. It is therefore not surprising that direct invasion of the left main bronchus by tumor is seen as a complication of advanced cancer of the middle third of the esophagus.

Understanding the appearance and MR signal characteristics of the esophagus and relations to nearby structures, such as the pleura, pericardium, azygos vein, and aorta, is essential for evaluation of potential surgical resection planes. In the treatment of patients with esophageal cancer, knowledge of the extent of tumor spread in relation to resection planes should facilitate preoperative surgical planning and identification of patients likely to benefit from neoadjuvant therapy.

SUMMARY

The esophagus is a unique and peculiar organ because it traverses the neck, the thorax, and the abdomen. Therefore, knowledge of its structure and anatomy is essential for any thoracic or general surgeon working in the area. Learning how to correlate the image with the anatomy is fundamental for the best surgical planning, not only for the indication but also for the potential difficulties. Because they are inexpensive and universally available, esophagograms should still be the first imaging examination of the esophagus. Although the esophagus is tubular and usually a flat structure, modern evaluation with a new generation of CT scans, MRI, and fiber-optic endoscopes offers precise and high-quality imaging.

REFERENCES

1. Hayward J. The lower end of the oesophagus. Thorax 1961;16:36–41.
2. Lang IM, Shaker R. Anatomy and physiology of the upper esophageal sphincter. Am J Med 1997; 103(5A):50S–5S.
3. Turco NB, Lemberg A, Hojman D. A note on the muscular structure of the lower third of the esophagus. Am J Dig Dis 1959;4:749–52.
4. Kalloor GJ, Deshpande AH, Collis JL. Observations on oesophageal length. Thorax 1976;31(3):284–8.
5. Friedland GW, Melcher DH, Berridge FR, et al. Debatable points in the anatomy of the lower oesophagus. Thorax 1966;21(6):487–98.
6. Schraufnagel DE, Michel JC, Sheppard TJ, et al. CT of the normal esophagus to define the normal air column and its extent and distribution. AJR Am J Roentgenol 2008;191(3):748–52.
7. Pope CE 2nd. The esophagus: 1967 to 1969. I. Gastroenterology 1970;59(3):460–76.
8. Bonavina L, Evander A, DeMeester TR, et al. Length of the distal esophageal sphincter and competency of the cardia. Am J Surg 1986;151(1):25–34.
9. Proto AV, Lane EJ. Air in the esophagus: a frequent radiographic finding. AJR Am J Roentgenol 1977; 129(3):433–40.
10. Pellegrini CA, Way LW. Esophagus and diaphragm. In: Way LW, editor. Current surgical diagnosis and treatment. Stamford (CT): Appleton & Lange; 1994. p. 841–53.
11. Castell DO. Anatomy and physiology of the esophagus and its sphincters. In: Castell DO, Richter JE, Boag D, editors. Esophageal motility testing. New York: Elsevier Science; 1987. p. 13–27.
12. Patti MG, Gantert W, Way LW. Surgery of the esophagus: anatomy and physiology. Surg Clin North Am 1997;77(5):959–70.
13. Skandalakis JE, Colborn GL, Weidman TA. Surgical anatomy: the embryologic and anatomic basis of modern surgery, vol. 1. Athens (Greece): Paschalidis Medical Publications; 2004.
14. Halber MD, Daffner RH, Thompson WM. CT of the esophagus: I. Normal appearance. AJR Am J Roentgenol 1979;133(6):1047–50.
15. Bowden RE, el-Ramli HA. The anatomy of the oesophageal hiatus. Br J Surg 1967;54(12):983–9.
16. Riddell AM, Davies DC, Allum WH, et al. High-resolution MRI in evaluation of the surgical anatomy of the esophagus and posterior mediastinum. AJR Am J Roentgenol 2007;188(1):W37–43.
17. Nakashima A, Nakashima K, Seto H, et al. Normal appearance of the esophagus in sagittal section: measurement of the anteroposterior diameter with ECG gated MR imaging. Radiat Med 1996;14(2):77–80.
18. Nakashima A, Nakashima K, Seto H, et al. Thoracic esophageal carcinoma: evaluation in the sagittal section with MRI. Abdom Imaging 1997;22(1):20–3.

FURTHER READINGS

Hagen JA, DeMeester TR. Anatomy of the esophagus. In: Shields TW, LoCicero J, Ponn RB, et al, editors. General thoracic surgery. 6th edition. Philadelphia: Lippincott Williams & Wilkins; 2005. p. 1885–93.

Kahrilas PJ. Functional anatomy and physiology of the esophagus. In: Castell O, editor. The esophagus. Boston: Little Brown; 1992. p. 1–27.

Libermann-Meffert D. Clinically oriented anatomy, embryology, and histology. In: Patterson GA, Cooper JD, Deslauriers J, et al, editors. Pearson's thoracic and esophageal surgery. 3rd edition. Philadelphia: Churchill Livingstone; 2008. p. 10–26.

Long JD, Orlando RC. Anatomy, histology, embryology, and developmental abnormalities of the esophagus. In: Feldman M, Friedman LS, Brandt LJ, editors. Sleisenger & Fordtran's gastrointestinal and liver disease: pathophysiology diagnosis/management. Philadelphia: WB Saunders; 2002. p. 551–60.

Index

Note: Page numbers of article titles are in **boldface** type.

A

Abdominal lymph trunks
    and thoracic duct, 230–233
Anatomy of the normal diaphragm, **273–279**
Anatomy of the pleura, 140, **157–163**
Anatomy of the pleura: reflection lines and recesses, **165–171**
Anatomy of the superior vena cava and brachiocephalic veins, **197–203**
Anatomy of the thoracic aorta and of its branches, **219–227**
Anatomy of the thoracic duct, **229–238**
Anatomy of the thymus gland, **191–195**
Aortic arch
    anatomy of, 220–222
    congenital abnormalities of, 222–226
Aortic hiatus
    and the diaphragm, 274–276, 278
Aortic valve
    anatomy of, 212–214
Aortopulmonary window
    on computed tomography, 269
Ascending aorta
    anatomy of, 219, 220

B

Basement membrane
    and the esophageal wall, 299–301
Brachiocephalic veins
    anatomy of, 198–202
    embryology of, 197, 198
    left, 198
    right, 198

C

Cardiac chambers
    anatomy of, 205–207
Cardiac plexuses, 246, 247
Central aponeurosis
    and the diaphragm, 273
Cervical esophagus
    computed tomography of, 313
Cisterna chyli
    and thoracic duct, 230–233
Congenital abnormalities
    double aortic arch, 225, 226
    Kommerell diverticulum, 223–225
    of the left aortic arch, 223, 224, 225

Coronary arteries
    anatomy of, 214–216
Coronary veins
    anatomy of, 216, 217
Correlative anatomy for the esophagus, **307–317**
Correlative anatomy for the mediastinum, **251–271**
Correlative anatomy of the diaphragm, **281–287**
Correlative anatomy of the pleura and pleural spaces, **177–182**

D

Descending thoracic aorta
    anatomy of, 226, 227
Diaphragm
    anatomy of, 273–279
    and aortic hiatus, 274–276, 278
    attachments of, 282, 283
    and attachments simulating pathologic processes, 283
    blood supply of, 274
    and central aponeurosis, 273
    configuration of, 281, 282
    correlative anatomy of, 281–287
    defects and areas of weaknesses, 283–287
    embryology of, 273
    and esophageal hiatus, 274–279
    imaging of, 281–287
    lymphatic system of, 274, 275
    muscular and tendinous portions of, 273, 274
    nerve supply of, 278, 279
    openings in, 275–278
    and phrenic arteries, 274
    and phrenic nerves, 273–274, 278, 279
    surface projection of, 152–155

E

Esophageal hiatus
    and the diaphragm, 274–279
Esophageal plexuses, 247, 248
The esophageal wall, **299–305**
    adventitia of, 303
    arterial supply of, 303
    and basement membrane, 299–301
    and epithelium, 299–301
    and lamina propria, 301
    lymphatic drainage of, 303, 304
    mucosa of, 299–302
    and muscularis mucosae, 301, 302

Thorac Surg Clin 21 (2011) 319–322
doi:10.1016/S1547-4127(11)00017-X

Moving?

Make sure your subscription moves with you!

To notify us of your new address, find your **Clinics Account Number** (located on your mailing label above your name), and contact customer service at:

Email: journalscustomerservice-usa@elsevier.com

800-654-2452 (subscribers in the U.S. & Canada)
314-447-8871 (subscribers outside of the U.S. & Canada)

Fax number: 314-447-8029

Elsevier Health Sciences Division
Subscription Customer Service
3251 Riverport Lane
Maryland Heights, MO 63043

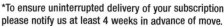

Moving?

Make sure your subscription moves with you!

To notify us of your new address, find your **Clinics Account Number** (located on your mailing label above your name), and contact customer service at:

Email: journalscustomerservice-usa@elsevier.com

800-654-2452 (subscribers in the U.S. & Canada)
314-447-8871 (subscribers outside of the U.S. & Canada)

Fax number: 314-447-8029

Elsevier Health Sciences Division
Subscription Customer Service
3251 Riverport Lane
Maryland Heights, MO 63043

To ensure uninterrupted delivery of your subscription, please notify us at least 4 weeks in advance of move.

Printed and bound by CPI Group (UK) Ltd, Croydon, CR0 4YY

03/10/2024

01040355-0011